Quick and Easy Medical Tips for Healthy Senior Living

Best wishes,

Sabeth Nower RN

Quick and Easy Medical Tips for Healthy Senior Living

Elizabeth Molle RN, MS

iUniverse, Inc.
New York Lincoln Shanghai

Quick and Easy Medical Tips for Healthy Senior Living

iUniverse, Inc.

For information address:
iUniverse, Inc.
2021 Pine Lake Road, Suite 100
Lincoln, NE 68512
www.iuniverse.com

ISBN: 0-595-31168-7

Creating a book from conception to publication requires strength and talent. My determination and strength came from my mother. My creativity and appreciation of the English language came from my Aunt Faith. I dedicate this book to the both of you. Thank you. I love you both very much. Betty

Contents

Preface

Graduation Day! My dream of becoming a Registered Nurse was fulfilled. The auditorium was packed. Clapping and cheering sounds could be heard for miles. No one clapped louder or cried more than my mom. Her dreams had also come true.

My nursing career has taken me on a path I never could have imagined. I worked as an emergency room nurse and then started teaching various medical courses. My yearning for patient care brought me back to work part time as a home care nurse. Wow! What an experience!

As a home care nurse, I witnessed first hand the trials and tribulations that you are experiencing. You are faced with daily concerns about your health and the future. Being admitted into a nursing home is a common fear among many older adults. My mother shares this fear with you. You can take steps to prevent this from happening. Be proactive. Plan for the future. You are in control of your destiny.

This book has been written to help you with those daily struggles. Each chapter focuses on a particular concern. Do not skip a chapter. It is the total package that will help you achieve the goal of independence.

You are not alone in this journey. There are answers to your questions. Resources are available for you and your family. Do not be afraid to reach out and grab them. Let the journey begin!

Introduction

Congratulations! You have taken the first step towards healthy senior living! This book will help you reach your goals. As the saying goes, "Lets get the ball rolling!" The two fundamental concepts you need to embrace include:

- Prevention is ninety-nine percent of the battle!
- Just go for it!

Prevention is ninety-nine percent of the battle! If you can prevent an injury or disease from knocking you down, you are ahead of the game. Prevention requires an aggressive approach to all aspects of your health. For example, if you have diabetes, you can take steps to prevent developing associated complications. If you have high cholesterol, you can take steps to prevent developing associated heart diseases. You will learn prevention tips in this book.

Just go for it! An offensive approach to life is better than a defensive one. Get up and go for it. Identify your goals and take action towards accomplishing them. Life is not easy. Growing older and developing health problems can seem overwhelming, frustrating, and even depressing. Do not let these issues take the wind out of your sail. You need to new find ways to motivate yourself.

Survey Results

According to a 2001 Gallup survey, the number one fear associated with old age is becoming a burden to family members or friends. You can prevent becoming a burden with preventive medicine and smart healthy living. *Do not let fear paralyze you; let it motivate you.*

In the same survey, nine out of ten people said they would prefer to be treated at home instead of a hospital or nursing home. You can live the rest of your life in your home, but it takes some preplanning. You need to create strategies to compensate for the changes that occur as you age. Learn about your healthcare needs and locate available resources.

Book Layout

Each chapter is divided into three sections. In the first section, "Just the Facts," you will find some important facts and information. Some interesting statistics are also included. Learn from them. *Do not let yourself become a statistic!*

In the second section, "Tip Exploration," you will find some practical every day tips. The tips are clearly marked in bold print. Implement as many tips as possible.

In the third section, "Internet Resources," you will find recommendations for Internet searching. If you do not have a home computer, you can:

- Go to your library, senior center, or community college.

- Highlight the sites you wish to search and bring this book to the library. Most librarians will be eager to assist you in searching the Internet.

Chapter one discusses the aging process and provides you with some tips for dealing with your body's changes. Chapters two through nine explore specific health care issues. Chapter ten answers some of the most frequently asked questions. There are five appendixes. Copy and use them at your doctor's appointments.

You will see two icons in this book: an owl and a key. The owl alerts you to a text box with some powerful words of wisdom. The key alerts you to a text box with important information about a specific health care issue.

This book is not intended to be a substitute for getting medical advice from a doctor or other health care professional. It is a supplement. Clarify information that is different from what your doctor has told you. People often say, "My doctor is too busy. I can not ask him questions." You are partially correct. *Doctor's work within tight time frames, but never be intimidated or leave an appointment unsatisfied with your plan of care.* Be organized when you go to the appointment. Use the appointment checklist in the back of the book. You and your doctor need to work together as a team.

If you feel still rushed at the doctor's office, ask for the last appointment of the day. If you have a specific illness, such as diabetes, ask for a referral to see a health care educator. An educator can spend more time with you and will answer all of your questions. Medicare will generally pay for these educational sessions.

1

The Aging Process: "What is Normal?" "What should I expect?"

Just the Facts

Aging is a beautiful transition that occurs in everyone's life. The body and mind are going through a variety of changes. These changes include body structure, financial, emotional, and spiritual. Some changes are pronounced and others ones are very subtle.

How old are you? This may seem like a simple question, but it is actually very complex. The answer is based on your chronological and physiological age. Chronological age refers to the number of candles on your birthday cake. It is merely a ceremonial number! Gerontologists sort chronological ages into four groups. The four groups are:

- Middle age (thirty-five to fifty-five years old).
- Advanced middle age (fifty-six to seventy-four years old).
- Aging (seventy-five to eighty-four years old).
- Elderly (eighty-five years old or older).

Physiological age refers to how well your body is changing. It takes into consideration your medical history, overall health, and activity level. Lets look at two different people and compare them.

- Barbara is fifty-five years old. She is twenty pounds overweight, has heart problems, and diabetes. She takes seven daily medications and is unable to climb a flight of stairs without stopping to rest.

1

- Paul is seventy-five years old and takes one medication to control his blood pressure. He jogs two miles per day and plays golf.

Chronologically Paul is twenty years older, but physiologically Barbara is much older. She takes more medications, is less active, and has more medical problems. She is not aging as well as Paul.

You may be saying, "men and women age differently anyways." The answer is yes and no. Men and women have the same physiological changes, but women have a longer life expectancy. A woman's life expectancy is seventy-nine years and a man's is seventy-four years.

You have the power to decide if you want to age like Barbara or Paul. Birthday candles are only symbols. *Do not act your age! Act the way you feel!* Enjoy life. Try new things. There is no age limit for hiking, swimming, or bike riding. If your mind says, "I can do it," then you will be able to do it. Believe in yourself.

The lifestyle you have lived for the past three or four decades will be factors in how well your body ages. A history of alcohol misuse, tobacco, steroids, or poor general health will accelerate the aging process. Multiple medical illnesses also accelerate the pace of aging. The good news is that today is a new day. You have the power to make changes, but it has to come from within you.

Genes also play a role in the aging process. Everyone has a special gene called Methuselah. It sits on the DNA chain and tells the body how fast to make certain changes. Researchers have not been able to slow the aging process, but with the identification of this gene it will happen someday!

What are the body's normal changes? Every part of the body goes through some normal changes. The most common body changes are described in the next few pages. If you know what body changes are normal, you can begin the process of acceptance. If something is not normal, you can begin to explore the cause and fix the problem. A simple example is memory loss. Old people are *not* always forgetful! Memory loss is a sign of a medical problem and its progression can sometimes be halted. Here is a look at the body's normal changes.

The Skin

Skin changes are the least dangerous, but they tend to bother us the most. Lines and wrinkles seem to appear overnight. You look in the mirror and suddenly reality sets in! The rate of skin changes is dependent on your diet, general health, genetics, and an accumulation of the sun's rays. Even one childhood sunburn will have an effect on the way your skin ages!

The most significant skin changes include:

- A flattening of the skin layers causing wrinkles and sagging to appear.

- A decrease in the blood flowing to the skin makes it more difficult for wounds and sores to heal.

- Collagen fibers become coarser causing less elasticity and more wrinkles.

- Melanocyte cell production decreases causing age spots to appear.

- Hair on the scalp, pubic, and axillary (armpits) becomes thinner and turns gray. Nasal and ear hair growth increases.

- Fingernails grow more slowly and become hard and brittle.

Pruritus (dry, itchy skin) is a common skin problem. Alleviate dry, itchy skin with creams and lotions. Be careful adding bath oils into the tub because it can make the surface slippery. Zinc oxide, which can be bought over the counter, can also help to control the dry, itchy feeling. Nutrition plays a huge role in keeping your skin healthy. Chapter four discusses nutrition in more detail.

Many creams advertise that they will tighten your skin and make you look younger. You may see some temporary changes, but in most cases they will not be permanent. Save your money!

The Heart

Each day your heart beats about one hundred thousand times and pumps about two thousand gallons of blood. The heart is a muscle and needs to be exercised. Unexercised muscles become weak. A weak heart pumps less effectively. The most significant heart changes include:

- Heart valves become thicker and do not operate as easily.

- Blood vessels become less elastic.

- Arteries and veins become narrower.

These changes make it harder for the blood to be pumped through the body. This causes the heart to work harder. If the heart is already weak, it is unable to keep the blood flowing adequately resulting in heart and breathing problems.

Most heart diseases can be controlled with diet, exercise, and good healthy habits. Follow your cardiologist's instructions and take medications as directed. Consider enrolling in cardiac rehabilitation classes. Medicare will cover the cost and most hospitals offer these programs.

High blood pressure (hypertension) is one of the most serious problems pertaining to the heart. The causes of hypertension include: various heart problems, genetics, stress, anxiety, and obesity. If you have hypertension, you need to take it seriously. Take your medications, lose weight, exercise, and follow your dietary instructions. *Uncontrolled hypertension can lead to life threatening problems.*

An estimated seven hundred thousand Americans will have a heart attack this year and about forty-two percent will die as a result of it. A heart attack occurs when the blood supply to the heart is stopped or reduced because of a blockage in the coronary arteries. The blockage is due to the buildup of plaque. Signs of a heart attack include:

- Chest pressure, tightness, or pain.
- Pain in the shoulders or the jaw.
- Trouble breathing.
- Nausea.
- Sweating.

If you think you are having a heart attack, sit down and call your local emergency services number. Do not attempt to drive yourself or a friend to the hospital. Time is muscle. More heart muscle can be saved when treatment is quickly started.

The Lungs

The most significant lung changes include:

- The rib cage becomes more rigid making it harder for the lungs to fully expand.
- The lung muscles become weaker and less effective.

- The lung tissue becomes less elastic making it harder to exhale carbon dioxide.

These changes make recovering from chest colds more difficult. It is harder for the body to remove chest congestion. A simple chest cold can easily turn into pneumonia.

If you have trouble breathing when walking short distances or climbing stairs, tell your doctor. This is not normal. Trouble breathing can be caused by heart or lung problems. Do not ignore the symptoms. *This is your life we are talking about!*

Great strides have been made in asthma management. If you have asthma and are dependent on an inhaler, see a pulmonologist. Newer medications are available. Ask your doctor for a spacer attachment. A spacer attachment helps to get the medication deeper into the lungs. You will be surprised with the results!

The Mouth, Stomach and Intestines

The most significant changes to these organs include:

- Teeth become more brittle and decay is more prominent.

- Less saliva is produced making swallowing more difficult.

- Slower stomach motility causes the stomach to take longer to empty.

- Less stomach acid is produced and fewer stomach cells can absorb nutrients.

- Stool moves through the colon more slowly resulting in constipation.

"Food does not taste the same. Nothing has any flavor." Does this sound familiar? Lack of taste is due to the changes in the taste buds. Look at your tongue. The bumps are called papillae. Each papilla holds about hundred taste buds. Taste buds allow the sensations of sweet, salty, sour, and bitter to be recognized. Umami, a recently identified taste bud, identifies the taste of monosodium glutamate. The average adult has about ten thousand taste buds.

The numbers of taste buds diminish with aging. Most people will lose about seventy percent of their taste buds by eighty years old. The taste buds left are less sensitive. The tastes from sweet and salty foods will be lost first. There are many ways to make food tasty again! Chapter four discusses this issue in more detail.

The Kidneys and Bladder

The two kidneys are located in the middle of the back. Kidneys are responsible for removing toxins and saving important electrolytes. The most significant kidney and bladder changes include:

- There is a reduction in the number of working kidney cells that makes filtering the toxins more difficult.
- The bladder begins to sag and holds less urine.
- Weaker bladder muscles increase the risk of acquiring bladder infections.

Drinking ample amounts of water will make your kidneys function better. Chapter five discusses urinating problems in more detail.

Urinary tract infections are the accumulation of the wrong bacteria in either the bladder or kidneys. The causes of urinary infections include: poor fluid intake, poor hygiene, and incomplete bladder emptying. Do not be alarmed if you develop a urinary tract infection following a hospitalization! Hospitals are breeding grounds for these infections.

The symptoms of a urinary tract infection include:

- An itchy, burning feeling after urinating.
- Urgency. This is a sensation of having to get to the bathroom fast.
- Frequency. This is a sensation of having to urinate, but you only go a small amount.
- Low grade fever.
- Lower backache.

If you experience those symptoms, get your urine tested. Do not delay. *A small urinary tract infection can quickly turn serious and require hospitalization.* Antibiotics are needed to treat urinary tract infections. You probably have heard that cranberry juice will cure a bladder infection. It will not cure it, but it will help to alleviate some of the symptoms and discomfort.

Take these steps to avoid getting urinary tract infections:

- Always wash your hands after using the bathroom.
- Completely empty the bladder. Sit on the toilet for an extra few seconds and rock back and forth. This will help to empty the bladder.

- Properly wipe yourself. Women should always wipe from front to back.

The Bones and Muscles

About two and half inches of body height is lost by eighty years old. The most significant bone and muscle changes include:

- The backbone discs become thinner and weaker causing the height loss.
- Back muscles become weaker causing a more stooped appearance.
- The tendons shrink making joint movement more difficult and painful.
- Cartilage in the weight bearing joints decreases causing hip and knee problems.

Osteoporosis is the loss of bone mass and a structural weakening of the bones. Fragile bones are more susceptible to breaking. About forty-four million Americans will develop osteoporosis and about eighty percent of its victims will be female. It can easily be detected with a bone density test. Most health insurance plans will pay for testing. Make your appointment today! Various treatment options are available for osteoporosis. *Stop its progression and maybe you can prevent breaking a bone!*

Arthritis is the inflammation of the joints. It is not possible to reverse the damages already present from arthritis, but you can take steps to control its progression. Keep your joints moving. Unused joints become stiff and eventually can not be moved.

A little exercise goes a long way towards being healthy. Chapter six discusses exercising in more detail.

The Brain

The most significant brain changes include:

- The number of active brain cells and the weight of the brain will decrease by about seventeen percent by seventy-five years old. *This reduction in brain cells and weight does not have an effect your thinking or behavior abilities.*
- Blood flow to the brain decreases.

- There is a reduction in the ability of your nerves to transmit impulses causing a slower response time, which can have an effect of your ability to safely drive a car.

Stroke is the one of the most life threatening brain illnesses. Strokes are the third leading cause of death in people over sixty-five years old. A stroke can cause minor problems or can result in major life threatening problems. Preventing a stroke from occurring is very important. High blood pressure is the number one risk factor for strokes. Get your blood pressure checked at least every six months. Most senior centers run free monthly blood pressure clinics. Supermarkets also have blood pressure machines, but these should only be used as screening tools. Their accuracy varies significantly. It is best is have your blood pressure checked by a health care professional. Write down your blood pressure readings and give it the doctor. Use a chart like this:

Date	Time	Blood Pressure	Comment
10/16	9:30 am	140/86	Taken at the senior center.
11/4	10 am	130/84	Taken at the supermarket machine
12/20	1 pm	160/102	Taken by my daughter after shopping all day

The Eyes

Changes to the eye will have an effect on your vision, primarily night time vision. The most significant eye changes include:

- The pupil size becomes smaller because the sphincter (type of muscle) in the eye hardens.
- A decreased blood supply to the eyes causes vision and depth perception problems.
- Floaters and cataracts often develop.

Floaters are caused by bits of debris that float in front of the lens. These floaters are not dangerous to your vision. *If you suddenly notice a change in your vision or total black out spots, call your doctor immediately or go to the hospital for an evaluation.* It can be a sign of a more serious problem.

Cataracts are common eye problems that occur when the lens loses its transparency. You have about a seventy percent chance of developing cataracts by seventy years old! Cataracts can appear in one or both of your eyes. They grow at different rates and cause vision to become distorted and blurry. Other symptoms include: poor vision in the sunlight, a milky appearance to the pupil, and an increased glare from oncoming car headlights. If left untreated, blindness will result in that eye. Doctors can diagnosis cataracts with an eye examination. A slit lamp may be used to see the cataracts exact location. Surgery is the primary treatment and usually is done as an outpatient procedure. You will be given antibiotics and steroid eye drops after the surgery. Recovery time is shorter and less difficult than years ago. A new eyeglass prescription can be issued within four to six weeks.

If you have cataracts, you should:

- Wear sunglasses.

- Use sheer curtains in your house to help to deflect the sunlight glare.

- Replace regular light bulbs with soft light bulbs.

The Ears

The most significant ear change is that the inner ear becomes harder and stiffer making hearing more difficult. High frequency noises and female voices are the hardest to hear. Sounds from letters *s, sh, f, ph, ch* are the most difficult. Do you have a hearing problem?

- Do you find yourself straining to understand people?

- Does everyone seem to be mumbling?

- Do you find yourself turning up the volume on the television or radio?

- Does your family ask you to turn down the volume on the television or radio?

- Do you have difficulty deciding what direction sound is coming from?

- Do you have trouble distinguishing certain familiar sounds?

If you answered yes to two or more questions, you should get your hearing tested.

Also, cerumen (ear wax) production increases. Ear wax traps dust and dirt particles before they can reach the eardrum. A build up of ear wax can be removed with a thorough ear cleaning. Before you get any ideas, stop and put down that cotton swab! *Never put anything smaller than your elbow into your ear!* Cotton swab devices should *only* be used to clean the outer part of the ear. You can buy ear drops to soften the wax. If you have ear pain, do not use these drops. Ear pain may be a sign of a perforated eardrum and using these drops can cause serious problems.

If you develop ringing in the ears, call your doctor especially if you are taking aspirin. High amounts of aspirin use can result in tinnitus. Your doctor will order blood tests to check the aspirin level. Tinnitus can also be caused by infections, hardening of the inner ear, or dental problems.

Debunking the Myths

These myths have been passed from generation to generation, but have been disproved by medical professionals. *Wash away these five myths:*

1. *Old people can not learn.* This is obviously not true. People who are intellectually challenged will have less memory loss and will be mentally sharper. Learn something new. Attend senior citizen classes, read a new book, meet new friends, or explore the Internet. Exercise your brain!

2. *Old people can not live alone.* You can live alone with proper care and planning. If you believe in yourself and are willing to accept help, you will remain independent. It depends on you and your motivation!

3. *Old people can not remember anything.* Nonsense! Your memory does not leave you because you turned seventy. Memory and cognitive changes are the result of a disease process. You need to seek medical attention to determine the root of the problem. Not everyone develops Alzheimer's. Alzheimer's is a disease that has become a catch phrase for person who forgets their car keys. If you or a loved one experiences a change in memory capabilities, get a professional evaluation.

4. *Old people can not be trusted to make financial and medical decisions.* You have the power to control your destiny. Never sign any legal papers unless you thoroughly understand what they say. Be open and honest with your family. Listen to their concerns. Estate laws change frequently. Chapter nine discusses various legal issues.

5. *Old people are always sick.* Older people are more likely to become sick and require hospitalization, but with proper care and preventive medicine you

are less likely to become sick. *Your doctor can not prevent diseases alone. You need to take the initiative to prevent getting sick.*

The Total Picture

You have learned about the physical changes and have erased the myths. You are now ready to start learning some new information. Below is your first set of tips. *These tips are some of the most important ones in the book.* Set a goal of trying two tips per day. Some tips will seem very obvious and basic, but they work. Prevention is the number one goal. If you can prevent an illness or injury, you are on the road to success!

Tip Exploration

Tip 1. Get a good doctor. A primary care doctor is someone who treats your every day problems. You should not use your gynecologist, cardiologist, or dermatologist to treat every day medical problems. These doctors are called specialists. Use an internist or a family practice doctor for regular examinations. If you only have a specialist, ask them for a referral. The local hospital may also have a doctor referral line.

A nurse practitioner is a registered nurse who has received special training and certification. They generally work with doctors and see patients in an office setting. They can perform physical examinations, order special tests or studies, and write prescriptions. If you are looking for a female doctor and are unable to find one, a nurse practitioner may be a great alternative!

Walk in centers, clinics, and emergency rooms should *not* be used for every day medical care. If you go to an emergency room for routine medical care, your insurance may not pay for the visit.

Write down the name of your primary care doctor: _____

Tip 2. Make an appointment to see the doctor, dentist, eye doctor, and hearing specialist. Plan a preventive medicine appointment today. Do not wait until you are sick. Some problems may go undetected until it is too late to fix them and permanent damage has occurred.

Appointment made to see your primary doctor: _____

Appointment made to see your dentist: _____

Appointment made for an eye examination: _____

Appointment made for a hearing test: _____

Put a √ here when done.

Tip 3. Learn from your past. Your family history provides clues for the future. Ask yourself, "What medical problems did my parents have?" If they had diabetes or heart problems, you are at a higher risk for developing these problems. Do not put your head in the sand. Be aggressive and proactive.

Tell your children about their grandparents' and great-grandparents' medical histories. Consider genetic counseling. For example, the gene linked to colon cancer has been identified. If two or more linear relatives had colon cancer, you can have a blood test done to look for the gene. Some insurance plans pay for genetic testing.

Tip 4. Allow extra time to gather thoughts and plan your day. Rushing to complete a job or project is asking for trouble. Things always take longer than you anticipate. Your reaction time is slower. If a project used to take ten minutes to complete, accept the fact that now it may take fifteen minutes. Getting mad or frustrated serves no purpose. Just plan accordingly.

Tip 5. Be open to change. Doing something the same way for the past ten years does not make it productive or safe. Be receptive to change. Do not become stubborn. Listen to suggestions and ideas. New and better appliances are available. Replace older appliances with new energy efficient ones.

Tip 6. Do not say the word "never!" Only you can make your dreams come true. If you have dreamed about traveling, learning something, or finishing school, go out and do it. You have the power to make those things happen. Certain medical problems may make it harder, but you have to take the first few steps. It is very easy to get sad and upset over life's problems. *View your problems as challenges.* If you view something as a problem, it will become one. Problems are hard to fix. If you view something as a challenge, you will be motivated to overcome it.

Depression is a very common illness. Your life has changed. You will never be thirty years old again and carefree. However, this does not mean that your life is over and you should throw in the towel! If you think you may be depressed, talk to a health care professional. Maybe you have built-up anger inside you that needs to be released or a ghost from your past needs to be set free. Face your problems and admit to your weaknesses. It is actually healthy.

Tip 7. Get a medical alert tag. If you have any of these medical problems, you should wear a medical alert tag: diabetes, cancer, seizures, heart condition, allergy to bees or any medications. They can be bought in most pharmacies. More stylish tags can be ordered through various companies and jewelry stores. Medical professionals can locate bracelets or necklaces styles the quickest.

Medical alert tag obtained. _____

Put a √ here when done.

Tip 8. Create an emergency card for your wallet. Emergency room personnel must have a quick and accurate medical history from you. Create an emergency medical card for your wallet. Include the following information:

- Your primary doctor's name. If you have specialists, include their names.

- A list of your medical problems. (Diabetes, cancer, high blood pressure).

- A list of your previous surgeries. (Gallbladder removed, appendix removed).

- A list of your medications. Include the medications name and dosage.

- A list of any allergies to medications.

- List any implanted medical devices. (Pacemakers, defibrillators).

- If you have had an angioplasty (balloon) or open-heart surgery, write down the part of the heart that was treated.

- If you have had a transplant, write the name of the organ and when the transplant was done.

- If you are on a transplant waiting list, write the name of the organ and the company or hospital that is searching for that organ.

Keep a list of contact names in your wallet. Your list should have at least two contact names and include this information: their full name, complete street address, telephone numbers (home, work, cellular), and pager numbers.

Emergency wallet card created. _____

Put a √ here when done.

Tip 9. Keep on moving. A good exercise program is essential. Exercise your heart and your brain. It is important to talk with your doctor before starting any exercise program. Start slowly and increase intensity as your body adjusts. Chapter six discusses exercising in more detail.

Tip 10. Make cheat notes! If you find yourself trying to remember things, make yourself cheat notes. Buy papers with sticky backs and post special notes in key areas. Write down phone numbers of important people and place them by the telephone. *Write down your telephone number on the sheet as well.* Sound silly? How often do you call yourself? If you do not use a number over and over again, you will forget it. It happens to everyone.

Tip 11. Drink plenty of fluids especially water. Dehydration is a leading cause of hospital admissions. Water helps the skin, heart, lungs, and kidneys to function. You lose water through urine, bowels, salvia, sweat, physical activity, and breathing! Water accounts for about fifty to seventy percent of your body's weight. Do not wait until you feel thirsty to drink water. Thirst is a warning sign from your body that you are low on fluids. *Try to drink six to eight glasses of water per day*. Soda, coffee, teas are not substitutes for water. If you live in a warm climate with high humidity, you must drink more water. If you live in a cold environment, drinking water will keep your body warmer. Why? Hydrated fat cells provide better and fuller insulation.

Tip 12. Apply sunscreens and wear broad rim hats when working in the yard. Decreased melanocyte production will increase your chances of getting sunburned. Certain medications also increase your body's sensitivity to the sun. If your medication bottle says, "This medication can cause photosensitivity," take it seriously. You will burn crisper than a potato in hot oil! Skin is the body's first line of defense. Protect it as much as possible. Plan outside activities during early morning or late afternoon hours.

Internet Resources

- Go to the National Library of Medicine (www.medlineplus.gov) web site for information about numerous medical illnesses.

- Go to the American Heart Association web site (www.americanheart.org) web site for information on recognizing, preventing, and treating both strokes and heart attacks.

- Go to the National Institute on Aging (www.nia.nih.gov) web site for information about aging and various resources for you and your family.

- Go to the National Institute on Health (www.nihseniorhealth.gov) web site for information about healthy senior living.

- Go to the American Medical Association (www.ama-assn.org) web site for help finding a doctor in your area.

- Go to a search engine and type these words: aging, preventive medicine, medical alert bracelets.

2

Home Safety:
"What can I do to prevent falling and breaking my hip?"

Just the Facts

Here are some stunning statistics about falls and the resulting injuries:

- Approximately one third of all people over sixty-five years old will fall each year.

- One third of all falls result in a serious injury reducing mobility and independence.

- Injuries from falls costs Medicare about thirty-five billion dollars a year.

- Two thirds of all falls occur at home and are from a standing height.

- According to the American Academy of Orthopedic Surgeons, one out of every seven women will break their hip!

The most common broken bones are the hip, back, and forearms. *Broken hips are one of the leading causes of nursing home admissions.* You can not prevent all falls, but you can take steps to decrease your risk.

What is a broken hip? A broken hip is a fracture of the thighbone. The thighbone (femur) is the largest bone in the body and supports your weight when walking or standing. Treatment for a broken hip depends on where the break is located. A femoral head fracture (break that is one to two inches below the hip joint) is fixed with pins. The tip of the thighbone may also be replaced with a metal ball. An intertrochanteric fracture (break that is three to four inches below the hip joint) is fixed with screws and a plate. Treatment also depends on your health and activity level.

Safety Tips

This set of tips focuses on safety. Some tips will seem very obvious and simple, but they are solid and effective. The goal is teach you ways to prevent falling and breaking bones. Swallow your pride and try these tips!

Tip Exploration

Tip 13. Change your position slowly. Sudden position changes, sitting to standing, can cause your blood pressure to suddenly drop resulting in a loss of balance. Dangle your feet off the edge of the bed before standing. After a long car ride open the car door and dangle your feet before standing. If you feel dizzy with sudden position changes, tell your doctor. He will check your blood pressure both sitting and standing and adjust your medications.

Tip 14. Wear shoes with laces and solid soles. Sneakers offer more traction and prevent falls better than shoes. Avoid high heeled shoes and open toed sandals. Wear slippers inside the house. If you have trouble knotting shoelaces, try Velcro laced shoes or elastic band shoelaces. (Elastic band shoelaces can be found in children shoe departments. They do not require tying and simply snap tight). It is safer to use these options than to walk with your shoes untied.

Tip 15. Obtain walking devices (canes, walkers) to help you. Walkers and canes are assistive devices. They increase your stability and help prevent falls. Use these devices correctly otherwise they can become a hazard. Chapter seven discusses these devices in more detail.

Tip 16. Ask your doctor about medications to improve your balance and walking. A fear of falling can cause more trouble with your balance than an actual physical problem. Medications can help eliminate the fear of falling and improve your balance. Express your concerns to the doctor. *Doctors can not write a prescription for something if they do not know that it is a problem.*

Some medications can actually increase your fall risk. Be aware of the side effects to your medications including: dizziness, drowsiness, dips in your heart rate, and drops in blood pressure. Sleeping pills and blood pressure medications have many of these side effects. Chapter three discusses medications in more detail.

Tip 17. Keep areas brightly lit, but avoid glare. Fluorescent lights produce glare. Two or three smaller lights scattered in a room will produce less eyestrain and less glare than one large bright light. Sunlight can be intrusive and can also produce glare. Use sheer curtains to block the sun's rays.

Be prepared for power outages and no indoor lights. Keep flashlights in your kitchen, bedroom, and basement. Be sure to keep spare batteries for the flashlights.

Tip 18. Keep your hot water heater at 110° F (43° C) degrees. The three reasons to lower the temperature on your hot water heater include:

- Hot water in the tub or sink can cause burns. Burns occur because the nerves are not as sensitive and the brain takes longer to interpret the hot sensations.

- Hot shower water can cause the blood pressure to drop because of vasodilatation. Vasodilatation is the opening or dilation of your arteries and veins.

- Lowering the hot water heater temperature will save you money!

Hot water heater temperature checked. _____

Put a √ here when done.

Tip 19. Install smoke detectors and carbon monoxide detectors. You should have a minimum of one smoke detector and carbon monoxide detector on each floor of your house. Change the batteries twice a year. Do not climb on a step stool or ladder to change the batteries. Ask a neighbor or family member for assistance.

Smoke and carbon monoxide detector installed. _____

Put a √ here when done.

Tip 20. Choose the best floor covering. Selecting the best flooring for your house depends on your personal taste, finances, and health. Consider these points:

- A shuffling gait on a rug will collect static electricity and can result in falling.

- Carpeting is difficult for wheelchair mobility and for cleaning.

- Scatter rugs can cause you to trip and should be eliminated.

- Tile flooring can be slippery and cold.

- If you are installing new linoleum or vinyl flooring, select a simple pattern. Complex patterns and bold colors can cause dizziness.

- Use nonskid flooring in the bathroom.

Tip 21. Avoid climbing stairs. Climbing stairs poses a safety hazard. If you do climb stairs, keep your hands empty. Never carry boxes up the stairs because they can disrupt your balance. Use the handrails. Do not put items on the stair steps to "be taken up" later. Instead put these items on a table next to the stairs.

Kitchen

Tip 22. No climbing on step stools! Rearrange cabinets to prevent the need for step stools. There is no such thing as a safe and sturdy stool. Prevention is the number one goal.

Tip 23. Never use the oven or stove to heat your house. Heating your house with a gas or an electric stove is very dangerous. If you lose power, go to a local shelter or senior center.

Tip 24. Change your kitchen sponges at least once a month. Kitchen sponges harbor nasty bacteria that can make you sick. Bacteria grow well in sponges because it is a moist and warm environment.

Date you changed your kitchen sponges: _____

Tip 25. Replace your old knives with sharp new ones. You are more likely to cut yourself using a dull old knife than a sharp new one. Ask for knives as gifts or start to replace them one at a time.

Bedroom

Tip 26. Do not smoke in bed. There are about three hundred thousand house fires every year. A death from a fire occurs about every one-hundred and seventy minutes. *According to the National Fire Protection Agency, smoking is the leading cause of house fires and adults over the age of sixty-five are at twice the risk of dying in a house fire.*

Tip 27. Clear the hallway to the bathroom before going to sleep. A night stand in the hallway is asking for trouble. Do not take a chance on remembering its location. Move it before you trip!

Tip 28. Keep a telephone by the bedside. Rushing to answer the telephone at two in the morning is not safe. Place a telephone near your bedside. Most telephone companies will install a phone jack at a reasonable price.

Bathroom

Tip 29. Install grab bars in the shower stall and near the toilet. Grab bars are inexpensive and can be purchased in local hardware stores. Ask the store clerk if they can recommend someone to install them.

Tip 30. Get a raised toilet seat. Do you find it difficult to pull yourself up to a standing position from the toilet? Try a raised toilet seat. You can purchase plastic toilet seat risers in most pharmacies. Do not pull yourself up using the towel rack or toilet paper holder. They are not built to support your weight.

Tip 31. Use a shower chair instead of standing while showering. A shower chair is placed inside the shower stall or tub and allows you to sit while showering. Install a handheld shower attachment for easier bathing while sitting. Handheld shower attachments also make cleaning the tub easier because they require less bending and straining.

Outside

Tip 32. Get motion sensor lights. These lights serve as a security alert and provide outside night time lighting. Two benefits for the price of one! Buy solar powered ones for easy installation.

Tip 33. Know your limits. Mowing the lawn, shoveling snow, and raking leaves are hard physical activities. Consider hiring an outside helper. Avoid climbing the ladder to clean the gutters. I have seen many broken bones from people climbing ladders. Every one of those patients said the same thing you are saying right now, "I have done it this way for the past thirty years and I have never gotten hurt!" Be smart. Prevention is the number one goal.

Tip 34. Keep walkways clear of obstacles including snow, ice, and leaves. Do not put flower boxes on the pathway into the house. Instead use hanging style flower boxes. Get broken steps replaced. Make sure the railings are secure and replace them as needed. Consider installing a ramp.

Unfortunately many unscrupulous people prey on older Americans. Do not let yourself become a victim to a senior predator. They will promise you anything and often appear very trustworthy and sincere. Do not let strangers into your house. If someone arrives at your door uninvited and says, "I am from the phone company and I need to see the inside phone lines," do not allow them inside until you contact the phone company. Never give your social security, checking, or credit cards numbers out over the telephone unless you have placed the call. Create an email address that does not use your full name. Use your initials or a fictitious name. Use caution when purchasing items online.

Internet Resources

- Go the National Center for Injury Prevention and Control (www.cdc.gov/ncipc) web site for information about injury prevention for all ages. The site is very easy to search.

- Go to American Academy of Orthopedic Surgeons (www.aaos.org) web site or call 1-800-824-BONES for a fall prevention brochure.

- Go to the National Fire Protection Agency (www.nfpa.org) web site for tips on fire safety and fire prevention.

- Go to a search engine and type these words: fall prevention, home safety, and fire safety.

Remember these key points when reading information on the Internet:

- Watch out for phrases like breakthrough, medical miracle, and secrete formula.

- Avoid sites advertising that they have "cured" a disease.

- Use caution when you see the phrase "ancient remedy."

- Use caution when you find a site that will treat a whole list of diseases with the same treatment.

- Do not believe every testimonial that you read.

- If the site claims that the government is hiding information to cure a disease, use extreme caution.

- Use caution when the treatment can "only be bought here."

- If the site says or alludes to "do not tell your doctor about this," stay away from the site.

- Go to www.quackwatch.com for a web site full of information about various health care frauds, fads, myths, and fallacies. Quackwatch is a nonprofit corporation.

- Send complaints to Federal Trade Commission www.ftc.gov about sites that provide information that is misleading and wrong.

3

Medications: "What should I do with all of these pills?"

Just the Facts

Eighty-four billion health care dollars is spent annually on medication related problems. *The failure to take medications properly results in ten percent of all nursing home admissions and an estimated twenty-five percent of all emergency room visits.* If you are admitted to the hospital as a result of a medication problem, your admission will be about four days longer. The average older person takes four prescription medications and two over the counter medications per day! *Medications can be a prescription for disaster unless you learn as much as you can about them.*

Medications are organized into groups based on how they work. The most common groups of medications are described below.

Analgesic Medications

Analgesics relieve aches and pains. Pain is a symptom of a problem. It is important to find out what is causing the pain. Analgesics alleviate the pain, but will not fix the underlying problem. Assume that you have a toothache. You can take an analgesic and the pain will go away, but the cause of the toothache will remain. If the cause is an infection, the infection will continue to grow and get worse. Take the analgesic and simultaneously seek medical attention to get rid of the cause of the pain.

Take analgesics as directed. Do not take more than the recommended dose. It can be dangerous. Do not drive or operate machinery, sign legal papers, or drink alcohol while taking analgesics.

Narcotics are a special type of analgesics. Here are three important tips about narcotics:

- They can be habit forming. If you have been taking narcotics for a prolonged time, you may experience withdrawal symptoms when stopping. Speak to your doctor before stopping any long term narcotic use.

- They can cause constipation. If you develop constipation, take a stool softener.

- They can cause stomach upset so take these medications with food.

Try to alleviate pain without medication. Consider these options: acupuncture, therapeutic touch, guided imagery, reflexology, and aromatherapy. Ask your doctor for a recommendation. Most doctors are willing to discuss alternative medicine therapies.

Antibiotic Medications

Antibiotics treat infections. They do not work on viruses and that is why your doctor will *not* prescribe antibiotics for the common cold. Overuse of antibiotics causes your body to develop resistance to them. If you are taking an antibiotic, it is essential that you finish taking the whole prescription.

Does this sound familiar, "You start taking an antibiotic and two days later you feel better, so you stop taking it?" This process is the culprit to the creation of "super bugs." A super bug is a mutated bacterium that is difficult and sometimes impossible to treat with traditional antibiotics.

Antibiotics can cause stomach upsets. If you develop diarrhea or stomach upset, call your doctor and he will prescribe a different antibiotic. Throw away the remainder of that antibiotic. Do not give it to your spouse or neighbor.

Antibiotics can cause allergic reactions. The signs of an allergic reaction include: hives, rash, tightness in the throat, and trouble breathing. If you experience those symptoms, call your emergency services number. Allergic reactions are life-threatening emergencies.

Some antibiotics should be to taken before meals while others need to be taken after meals. Food can have an effect on the ability of the antibiotic to get absorbed into the blood stream. Follow the instructions on the prescription bottle carefully.

Anti-inflammatory Medications

Anti-inflammatory medications control inflammation and swelling. The swelling can be anywhere in your body, but usually is in the joints or muscles. These medications can cause stomach irritation. Signs of stomach irritation include: pain, nausea, loss of appetite, and heartburn. If you have a sensitive stomach or history of bleeding in the stomach, speak with your doctor before taking any anti-inflammatory medications.

Long term use of certain anti-inflammatory medications can cause kidney and liver problems. Tell your doctor how often you are taking any over the counter anti-inflammatory medications. He may prescribe a better medication that has fewer side effects.

Anticoagulant Medications

Anticoagulants thin the blood. "Thinning the blood," means that the blood will run through the arteries and veins easier. It changes the bloods ability to form clots. These medications are prescribed for certain heart problems and for dissolving blood clots. If a blood clot is left alone inside the body, it can become dislodged and travel. *A traveling blood clot is very serious.* It may land in your heart, lungs, or brain and can result in death or other serious injuries. If you are taking a blood thinner, it is very important to have routine blood tests done to monitor your body's ability to form clots. Too much of this medication is not a good thing!

Follow the dietary restrictions your doctor or pharmacist gave you. If you did not get a list of foods to avoid, call your pharmacist and he will provide you with one. Green leafy vegetables are the main food concern. If you enjoy eating green leafy vegetables, eat a consistent amount so that your medication level can be altered to meet your body's needs.

Coumadin, a common anticoagulant, interacts with many medications. Do not take any herbal supplements or over the counter medications unless you have reviewed them with your pharmacist. Avoid alcoholic beverages when taking Coumadin.

Lovenox, another common anticoagulant, is given by injection. If you are taking this medication, follow the instructions in the packet for correct sites and techniques. Rotate your sites and keep a record of site selection.

Always take anticoagulants the same time each day. Most doctors advise patients to take these medications in the afternoon so that dosages can be adjusted following blood work results.

If you fall and hit your head while taking an anticoagulant, go to your local emergency room for an evaluation. You may initially feel fine, but you could develop a small bleed or hemorrhage.

Contact your doctor immediately if you notice these things:

- Bright red blood in your urine.

- Bright red blood in your stools or dark tarry stools.

- Bleeding from your nose or gums.

Antihypertensive Medications

Antihypertensive medications control high blood pressure. High blood pressure is known as the silent killer because it causes strokes, heart attacks, and kidney damage without warning. A blood pressure consists of two numbers and is written as a fraction (for example, 120/82). The upper number is called systolic and tells the doctor how much force is on the heart when it pumps blood. The lower number is called diastolic and tells the doctor how much force is on the heart at rest. The acceptable ranges for your blood pressure are determined by your medical condition, age, and existing illnesses.

In May 2003, the American Heart Association released a new study that has changed the way doctors treat high blood pressure. A systolic reading of greater than one hundred and forty requires treatment regardless of the diastolic reading in people over fifty. Prior to this study doctors worried more about the bottom number than the top.

Fifty million Americans will develop hypertension during their lifetime. Are you one of them? If you have not had your blood pressure checked within the last six months, you should get it done.

It is never "ok" to stop taking antihypertensive medications without your doctor's permission. Do not self adjust the medications based on a blood pressure reading at a local clinic. Your blood pressure is "ok" because you are taking the medication!

Antihypertensive medications can cause dizziness with any sudden position change. Change your position slowly. Dangle your feet on the side of the bed before getting up or standing. Report any dizzy episodes to your doctor.

Some antihypertensive medications will have an effect on your blood sugar. If you are diabetic and are starting a new antihypertensive medication, test your blood sugar daily for at least two weeks. If your blood sugar levels increase, call the doctor.

Some antihypertensive medications will have an effect on your potassium level. Ask the pharmacist if your medication changes potassium levels and follow their instructions regarding potassium supplements.

If you use salt substitutes to control your sodium level, be aware that they contain potassium. High levels of potassium can lead to irregular heart rhythms. Do not over use salt substitutes.

Cholesterol Lowering Medications

Cholesterol lowering medications help control the amount of plaque in your arteries. Plaque can cause a blockage of blood. When the blockage occurs, the blood can not get to the muscle and the muscle dies. Plaque can also become loose and travel in the arteries. Traveling plaque can land in your brain or heart resulting in a stroke or heart attack.

Routine liver function blood tests will be required while taking these medications. These medications are dissolved in the body's liver and can lead to liver problems if not closely monitored.

Your doctor prescribed this medication because your blood cholesterol levels were too high. Medications can only lower your cholesterol by only so much. You need to make dietary changes. *There is no such thing as a magic pill!*

These medications tend to be very expensive, but as the patents expire the cost will come down. Ask your doctor for free samples and request generic brands if available.

Diabetic Medications

Diabetes management consists of various types of medications. Diabetes is a chronic, long term disease that is treated with diet, exercise, and medications. If you do not properly care for your diabetes, it can lead to many complications. Some of the most serious complications include: heart attacks, strokes, poor leg circulation, delayed wound healing, and even blindness. *If you take an aggressive, preventive approach to your diabetes, you can avoid those complications.*

Numerous medications are available to control diabetes. Initially you will be started on oral medications and diet control. If your diabetes can not be controlled with this combination, you will be started on insulin. Insulin is given as a daily injection. Whether you are taking oral or insulin medications, you should test your blood sugar on a regular basis. This can be done with a simple finger stick in privacy of your house. Ask your doctor for a referral to see a diabetes educator. Your diabetes will not just go away. You need formal teaching about diet, exercise, and managing your blood sugars.

Diuretic Medications

Diuretics help the body flush away extra fluid. Extra fluid accumulates in your legs, heart, and lungs causing problems. Once the extra fluid is removed you will feel better. Diuretics can also help control your blood pressure.

Diuretics can cause the body to lose important electrolytes, such as, potassium, sodium, and chloride. Eat well-balanced meals and keep your body hydrated when taking them. If you develop diarrhea, contact your doctor. Diarrhea causes you to lose the same electrolytes. *If you lose too many electrolytes, it can be very dangerous.*

Gout Medications

Gout is an illness caused by high uric acid levels in the blood. The uric acid forms crystals that become trapped in your joints and causes pain. There are two types of gout medications. One type is used for acute or sudden attacks and the other is used to prevent recurrent attacks.

If you are taking a gout medication to prevent recurrent attacks, never stop taking this medication unless advised to by the doctor. A sudden stoppage can trigger a severe gout attack. Gout medications are a life long treatment.

The most common side effects from gout medications are easy bruising, bleeding, and rashes. If you notice big black and blue bruises after only a small injury, talk to your doctor. The dosage may need to be readjusted. If you develop a rash, call your doctor and he will change your medication.

If you have gout, follow a low purine diet. A low purine diet limits these foods: meats, anchovies, liver, sardines, kidneys, lentils, sweet breads, and peas. Alcohol and excessive aspirin use may also trigger gout attacks.

Heart Medications

Three common types of heart medications include: nitroglycerin, blockers, and digoxin. Nitroglycerin is a vasodilator. It opens the blood vessels allowing blood to flow easier. Nitroglycerin is used to control angina pain. Angina is caused when the arteries in your heart become tight and constrict. Nitroglycerin opens the arteries resuming blood flow and thus the pains go away. If the pain does not go away, you need to call your local emergency service number and go the emergency room.

Blockers regulate your heartbeat and keep it within a safe range. The two types of blockers are calcium channel and beta blockers. Never stop taking these pills without checking with your doctor. It can be very dangerous.

Digoxin increases the force of your heart's contractions. It makes your heart pump better and more effectively. If you are taking digoxin and notice any vision changes, muscle spasms, or weaknesses, you need to call your doctor. A blood test will be ordered to check the drug level in your body.

Learn how to count your pulse. First, find the pulse in your neck or wrist. Count the pulsations for one minute. It should be between sixty and one hundred beats per minute. If you feel like your heart is racing or palpating in your chest, go to your local emergency room. If your pulse is less than fifty, call your doctor.

Hypnotic Medications

Hypnotics help you sleep better. If taken correctly, they are safe. Never attempt to drive a car or operate machinery after taking a hypnotic. If your bedroom is on the second floor, take the hypnotic after climbing the stairs.

Hypnotics should only be used as a short term therapy. They are *not* meant to be a permanent solution to a sleeping problem. Take the smallest dosage possible.

Try these tips for better sleeping:

- Play soft music in the bedroom.
- Have a glass of warm milk before bedtime.
- Avoid napping during the day.
- Go to bed at a regular time each night.
- Do not allow yourself to fall asleep on the couch watching television. It is a bad habit!

🔑 You may be taking sleeping pills because of an undiagnosed medical problem. You may have sleep apnea. Sleep apnea is a disruption in the breathing pattern while sleeping. Periods of irregular breathing last about ten seconds, but can occur as often as thirty times per hour! The signs of sleep apnea include: heavy snoring, struggling to breathe during sleep, suddenly being awoken by a loud snort, and a feeling of excessive tiredness during the day even after "sleeping" all night. Most hospitals have sleep clinics that can diagnosis and treat these problems. Every one needs a restful sleep!

Laxative Medications

Laxatives help to alleviate constipation, however, they are often misused and over used. Overuse of laxatives can lead to serious problems. Regulate bowel movements with good dietary habits. Chapter five discusses constipation in more detail.

Thyroid Medications

The thyroid hormone has many functions, including:

- Keeping the muscles strong.
- Promoting metabolism.
- Giving you energy.
- Helping to control your weight.
- Keeping your skin healthy.
- Keeping your memory sharp.
- Helping to regulate your heartbeat.

If your thyroid level is too low, you will need medications to increase your thyroid level. Common thyroid replacement medications are Synthroid or Levothyroxine sodium. *Take these medications the same time each day.* Take them before breakfast to help prevent insomnia, which is a common side effect. If you develop chest pain, tightness in your chest, palpitations, or shortness of breath while taking a thyroid hormone replacement, call your emergency services number. *Never change the brand of thyroid replacement medication without speaking to your pharmacist.* Variations in the dosage can be dangerous.

If your thyroid is over working, you will need to take a thyroid hormone antagonist. These medications help to lower the body's thyroid hormone level. If you take this type of medication, limit your iodine intake. Iodine can be found in salt, shellfish, and certain cough medications.

Urinary Continence Medications

Urinary continence medications control the over active bladder. Chapter five discusses the causes of urinary incontinence in more detail. Detrol is the most common over active bladder medication and has relatively few side effects. The most common complaint is dry mouth. It does not interact with any foods and very few medications. People with narrow angle glaucoma should *not* take this medication. Do not suffer or be embarrassed with a leaky bladder problem. Talk to your doctor and get treatment. You will feel much better!

Using This Information

Keeping medications organized and properly taking them can be an overwhelming task. Improperly taking medications may result in serious health problems and even death. Plus medications are expensive and you deserve the best possible results from them! Follow these tips to maximize medication results and to prevent problems.

Tip Exploration

Tip 35. Ask questions about your medications. Before taking any medication, you should ask these six questions:

- *What is the purpose of this medication? Why do I need to take it?* For example, is it going to control my blood pressure, diabetes, or my arthritis?

- *What dose of medication should I take?* Most medications are prescribed in milligrams, which is a metric measurement. The pharmacist is legally responsible for making instructions clear to you so that you know how many pills or how much liquid to take. For example, if the doctor prescribed fifty milligrams and each pill is twenty-five milligrams, the pharmacist should convert this to "take two pills". Do not engage in math exercises! Call your pharmacist for clarification.

- *How many times a day should I take it?* If the medication is to be taken more than once a day, it should be evenly distributed throughout the day. For example, if you need to take a medication twice a day, take one pill in the morning and the other pill about twelve hours later. If you are taking a medication three times a day, you should take one pill every eight hours.

- *What time of day should I take it?* It matters! Some medications need to taken in the morning while other medications need to be taken at bedtime.

- *What are the potential side effects of this medication?* A word to the wise: every medication has numerous potential side effects. Do not panic when you see the list, but be aware of them. The most frequent side effects are generally in italics or bold print. If you experience a side effect, call your doctor for additional instructions. Some medications can not be abruptly stopped.

- *Are there any foods that interact with this medication?* For example, grapefruit juice interacts with many antibiotics and some heart medications. Coumadin interacts with many foods. Food may slow the absorption of some medications and thus the medication must be taken on empty stomach. While other medications must be taken with food. It is best to take medications with water. Carbonated beverages or hot beverages can alter the covering of some medications.

Your pharmacist or doctor can answer the above questions. *The only stupid question is the one that you do not ask!*

Tip 36. Organize your medications. There are numerous ways to do this. Start the process by creating a medication chart. In the left hand column, write down the times of day that you need to take medications. On the top write the name of each medication you are taking. (I have listed four common medications as examples). Place a check mark in the appropriate columns. Make copies of this table and bring it with you to all of your doctor appointments.

	Digoxin (regulate heart beat)	Coumadin (blood thinner)	Azmacort (to help my breathing)	Ambien (sleeping pill)
Morning (8 am)	√		√	

	Digoxin (regulate heart beat)	Coumadin (blood thinner)	Azmacort (to help my breathing)	Ambien (sleeping pill)
Noon (12 noon)				
Dinner (6 pm)		√	√	
Bedtime (10 pm)			√	√

Pill boxes help to organize medications. They are inexpensive and can be purchased in most pharmacies. You can buy boxes with single time frames or boxes with multiple time frames. If you have arthritis, you may find single row boxes easier to handle and open. Ask your family to help fill the boxes.

Medication chart completed. _____

Put a √ here when done.

Be aware of fancy boxes and gadgets that are sold to handle your medications. You can buy boxes with alarms and flashing lights! Save your money to buy the medications you need. If the above tip does not help, speak to your doctor. Some medications can be ordered in longer acting preparations. This means you may only have to take the medication once a week instead of every day.

Tip 37. Buy all your prescriptions at one place. Most pharmacies have computerized programs that collect data about your medications and medical history. The computer cross checks your medications for interactions and disease contraindications. For example, a certain medication may be dangerous for people with asthma. The computer alerts the pharmacist who then calls the doctor and a safer medication is ordered.

Tip 38. Do not skip or double up on your medications. Medications should be taken within one hour of the prescribed time. If you forgot to take your medication and it is almost time for the next dose, take the next dose now. Do not double up on your medication. Doubling the dosage of certain types of medications can be dangerous.

Tip 39. Always finish your prescription. Many people take medications until they feel better and then stop. This can be very dangerous. Stopping some medications, such as a gout medication, can cause your body to have a rebound response and trigger an attack. Stopping a blood pressure medication may result in a stroke!

Tip 40. Alcohol interacts with some medications. When alcohol is combined with certain medications, more alcohol can enter the blood stream. For example, if aspirin is taken before a drink is consumed, more alcohol will be absorbed into the blood stream. Combining alcohol with other medications can increase your risk of liver damage. *Alcohol should never be taken with sleeping pills, tranquilizers, blood thinners, or antihistamines.* An occasional glass of wine can be safely consumed with other medications.

Tip 41. Supplements can be beneficial, but some are very dangerous. If you are taking supplements, tell your doctor. All herbal supplements must be stopped two to three weeks prior to surgery.

Do supplements work? You be the judge. You can read one study that says it will work and another study to say that it will not work. Here are the pros and cons of three common supplements:

- Garlic can prevent cancer and heart disease, but it increases your risk of bleeding.

- Ginkgo can decrease the symptoms of Alzheimer's disease and improve your memory, but it increases your bleeding time.

- Echinacea can help with flu or cold symptoms, but can be dangerous to people who have had a transplant (it can trigger a rejection) or people with autoimmune illnesses.

If you are going to use supplements, read the labels carefully. Talk to your pharmacist or doctor about any interactions with your medications. Buy supplements from your local pharmacy and make sure they carry the United States Pharmacopoeia (USP) bar code. The USP bar code means that the manufacturer has met certain safe manufacturing practices. *Do not assume it is safe because it is a natural product!*

Tip 42. Seek financial resources for buying medications. Most states have special programs for senior citizens that defer the cost of prescription medications. These programs are based on your income. Ask the pharmacist if they have senior discount days. Your prescription medications will not be covered, but you will be able to save money on the over the counter medications. If you have access to the Internet, search for the drug manufacturer (for example, Pfizer, Glaxo). Some manufactures offer special discounts for seniors. Doctors often receive free medication samples from drug manufacturers. Be assertive and ask for them!

Do not divide the dosage to save money. The medication dosage is based on your weight and the drugs therapeutic result. Some medications when taken in a lesser dosage can actually have a reverse action!

Try these other money saving tips:

- Ask for generic brand medications.

- Ask for your insurance company's drug formulary. A formulary is a list of medications that they accept. If the medication is not on the formulary, you may have to pay the total cost. Ask for a suitable substitute.

- Save all medication receipts and ask an accountant if you are eligible for medical tax deductions.

Tip 43. Use caution when buying medications on the Internet or from another country. Federal laws regulate both of these actions. These methods can save you money, but it can be illegal and dangerous. All United States pharmaceutical companies must follow strict safety and quality control measures. Other counties do not have the same strict rules or enforcement. The United States Food and Drug Agency (www.fda.gov/oc/buyonline) is an excellent web site for additional information on this topic. Check it out!

Tip 44. Get your blood tests done. Some medications require routine blood testing. Blood tests tell the doctor about any potential dangers. The most common blood tests look at your liver and kidney functioning. Other blood tests tell the doctor if the medication is working. For example, a blood test called hemoglobin A1C tells the doctor if your diabetes medication is properly working. If the medication is not properly working, the dosage can be changed or a new medication can be started.

Tip 45. Keep medications in the correct bottles. Do not use old bottles with incorrect labels. This is an accident waiting to happen! If you have a hard time opening regular bottles, ask the pharmacist for non-childproof containers. Be sure to keep these bottles away from small children.

Tip 46. Do not break or crush medication pills. Some pills can not safely be broken or crushed. Slow release and enteric coated medications can *not* be crushed. The pharmacist can tell you which medication pills can safely be broken.

Tip 47. Clean out your medicine cabinet! Throw away any prescribed medications that you are no longer taking. Do not save them. Check the expiration dates on all over the counter medications. Medications taken after their expiration date can be less effective and some actually become toxic. Prescription medications are generally safe for one year from the date the prescription was filled.

Internet Resources

- Go to the Medicare (www.medicare.com) web site for new information about its prescription drug benefit.

- Go to your state's department of health web site. Look for information about their drug assistance program.

- Go to the National Center for Complementary and Alternative Medicine www.nccam.nih.gov web site for more information on alternative medicine therapies.

- Go to the Safe Medication (www.safemedication.com) web site for information on taking your medications safely. It also has information on how to administer ear, eye, and suppository medications. You can type in the name of a medication and obtain information on that medication.

- Go to a search engine and type the name of your medication. Follow the link to the manufactures web site. Look for information about financial programs offered by that company.

4

Nutrition: "What should I eat?" "Why should I read the food labels?"

Just the Facts

Diet is a four-letter word that many people would rather not discuss, but we are what we eat. Think of food as your body's fuel. Just like putting gas into your car to make it run, you need to put food into your body to make it run. *The better the fuel, the longer and healthier mileage you will get from your body!* The need for good fuel becomes more important as you age. Eating healthy balanced meals will make you stronger. Eating meals full of sugar and fats will indirectly make you weaker.

Diet can increase the risk of acquiring and developing complications from these diseases: gout, cancer, anemia, diabetes, high blood pressure, high cholesterol, and heart disease. If you eat right, the progression of these diseases can be controlled and in some cases reversed. If you become sick, your body will not heal without proper nutrients. Being overweight or underweight can cause health problems. To stay healthy, you need to eat healthy.

Registered dietitians are the best resource for nutritional information. Ask your doctor for a dietitian referral. Depending on your medical condition, your insurance company may pay for the nutritional consultation. Dietitians can create tailored diet plans for you based on your medical conditions and food preferences.

Nutritional information can be very confusing. Start by learning to read food labels. The United States Food and Drug Administration mandates the information that must be on food labels. Food labels provide you with nutritional information about the food in that container. Food labels are also known as nutrition facts. Look at the sample nutrition facts label. Assume this label is for macaroni and cheese.

Nutrition Facts		
Serving Size 1 cup (228g) **Servings Per Container 2**		
Amount Per Serving		
Calories 400	Calories from Fat 100	
		% Daily Value
Total Fat 13g		20%
Saturated Fat 3.5g		23%
Trans Fat 2g		
Cholesterol 10 mg		3%
Sodium 500 mg		31%
Total Carbohydrates 48 g		16%
Dietary Fiber 2g		5%
Sugar 7g		
Protein 11g		
Vitamin A 15%	• Vitamin C 0%	
Calcium 15%	• Iron 15%	

Here is the bottom line!

↓

← **Stick to the serving size! Remember to double the numbers below if you eat more than 1 cup.**

← **No more than 30% of your total calories should come from fat!**

←**Less is best!**

← **Watch your sodium count, especially in prepackaged and canned foods!**

← **Try to eat 20-25 grams of fiber per day!**

← **You only need about 50 grams of protein per day!**

← **Get your vitamins from fresh fruit and vegetables!**

A nutrition facts label must include:

Serving Size: A serving size is the portion size. It can be listed in various measurements. For example, it may be listed as a slice, teaspoon, cup, or as pieces. In the food label example, one serving is a cup.

The serving size may or may not be appropriate for you depending on your weight, medical conditions, and what else you are eating at that time. If you eat double the serving size, you will need to double all the below numbers.

Servings per container: This line tells you how many servings are in the package. The sample label tells you there are two servings per container. This container has a total of two cups of macaroni and cheese.

Total Calories: Think of calories as the fuel for your body. Calories come from carbohydrates, fat, and proteins. The amount of calories your body needs depends on your age, height, weight, health, and activity level. If you consume more calories than your body needs, you will gain weight. If you consume fewer calories than your body needs, you will lose weight. The United States Food and Drug Administration along with the United States Department of Agriculture has set guidelines specifying what the average person needs for nutrition on a daily basis. These guidelines are called RDI (reference daily intake), previously called recommended daily allowances. The recommendation is based on the average adult person needing two thousand calories per day. You may need more or less than two thousand calories. Ask your doctor or dietitian how many calories per day you should consume. On the sample food label, there are four hundred calories in one serving.

Calories from Fat: This number tells you how many calories come from fat in one serving. *No more than thirty percent of your total food calories should come from fat*. In the food label example, there are one hundred calories from fat. In other words, about twenty-five percent of the calories are from fat!

Total Fat: Although fat is perceived as something bad, your body needs to consume some fat every day. Fat is needed for the body to grow and develop. It is also needed to transfer vitamins into the blood stream. The key is moderation. In the food label example, the total fat in one serving is thirteen grams. Based on a two thousand calorie diet, your daily fat intake should not exceed sixty-five grams. Therefore, in one cup of macaroni and cheese, you have eaten about twenty percent of your daily-recommended fat allotment.

Underneath the total fat is the **saturated fat content**. Saturated fat is the "clogging" material that causes health problems. Saturated fats increase your "bad" cholesterol, cause certain cancers, and can contribute to obesity. *Choose foods that have less than one-third of their total fat as saturated fat.* On the sample label, the saturated fat content is three and a half grams per serving. Based on a two thousand calorie diet, your saturated fat intake should not exceed twenty grams per day.

Trans Fat: Trans fat is a new requirement for food labels. Trans fats act like saturated fats. It raises your bad cholesterol, lowers your good cholesterol, and increases your chances of heart diseases. Trans fats are made when manufactures add hydrogen to cooking oils. This increases the products shelf life and keeps the taste stable. Major sources of trans fats include: snack foods, baked goods, salad dressings, processed foods, and fried foods. On the sample label, the trans fats content is two grams per serving. There are no formal limits on how many trans fats you should consume, but less is best. Food labels must list trans fats by January 1, 2006.

Cholesterol: Cholesterol is a soft waxy substance made by animals. Your body needs some cholesterol to work properly, however, your body is able to make what it needs. Cholesterol is found in foods that come from animals (beef, chicken, lamb, eggs) and from manufactured foods (crackers, chips, nuts).

The two types of cholesterol are low-density lipoprotein (LDL) and high-density lipoprotein (HDL). LDL is known as the bad one because it causes plaque to build up in your arteries. LDL also helps your cells to properly function. HDL is known as the good one because it helps remove some plaque from your arteries.

Your daily intake of cholesterol should not exceed three hundred milligrams. If you have heart disease or a high LDL level, the American Heart Association recommends that your total daily cholesterol level not exceed two hundred milligrams. On the sample label, the cholesterol content is ten milligrams per serving.

Eating vegetables and fruit will help lower your cholesterol. Eat meat and eggs in moderation. Food labels that say "cholesterol free" contain less than two milligrams of cholesterol per serving.

Sodium: Sodium is a component of salt. Salt contains about forty percent sodium and sixty percent chloride. Sodium makes your muscles contract and nerves react. Sodium can cause your body to retain fluids and thus increases your blood pressure. Limit your intake of sodium to two thousand four hundred milligrams per day. If you are sodium sensitive or have heart problems, you should keep your sodium level to less than two thousand milligrams per day. On the sample food label, the sodium content is five hundred milligrams per serving! That is one quarter of your daily allowance!

Limit your sodium intake by:

- Using frozen vegetables instead of canned.

- Avoiding smoked meats, sausages, processed foods, hotdogs, and bologna.

- Limiting snacks foods (chips, pretzels, crackers).

Replace the salt flavor with various spices, such as, dill, garlic, basil and bay leaves.

⌕ Sodium can be found in many items. For example, one tablespoon of ketchup has about one hundred and eight milligrams of sodium. A dill pickle has about eight hundred milligrams of sodium! One twelve ounce can of beer has about eighteen milligrams, but a twelve ounce can of club soda has about seventy-five milligrams of sodium. One buffered aspirin has about five hundred and fifty milligrams of sodium. The numbers are approximated because each company makes its product slightly different. Tally everything into your daily sodium intake.

Potassium: Potassium functions include: maintaining fluid balance, helping the nerves to transmit impulses, maintaining blood pressure, strengthening muscle contractions, and helping the heart to pump. Your body needs three thousand five hundred milligrams of potassium daily. You may need higher amounts if you are taking water pills (diuretics) or laxatives. Diarrhea and vomiting also causes your body to lose potassium.

Good potassium sources include: bananas, oranges, cantaloupe, and dried apricots and prunes. Vegetables that contain potassium include: broccoli, spinach, tomatoes, winter squash, baked potato, and Lima and pinto beans. Milk is also a good source of potassium.

Total Carbohydrates: Carbohydrates provide your body with energy. Your body breaks down carbohydrates into sugar. Total carbohydrates include: starches, simple sugars, and dietary fiber. *Your daily carbohydrate intake should not exceed three hundred grams.* On the sample food label, the carbohydrate content is forty-eight grams per serving.

Dietary Fiber: Fiber promotes bowel regularity, decreases the total blood cholesterol level, and lowers your body's LDL level. A good daily fiber intake reduces your risk of developing heart disease and colon cancer. *You should eat about twenty to twenty-five grams of fiber per day.* Most Americans fall short of this recommended level. On the sample food label, the fiber content is only two grams per serving.

Good fiber sources include: oats, flaxseeds, whole grain breads, prunes, brussell sprouts, and dried beans. Fruit skins (apple, pear, peach) are high in fiber content. Popcorn is another good source, but do not add butter or salt to the popcorn!

Sugar: The average American consumes over one hundred pounds of sugar per year. It is consumed through soda, candy, sweets, fruits, ice cream, and other dairy products. There is no daily maximum sugar amount you should consume, but less is better!

Protein: Protein builds and maintains muscle strength. It also helps your cells to function. *The average person needs about fifty grams of protein per day.* Long term diets high in protein can cause high blood pressure, kidney disease, and bone density loss.

Good protein sources include: nuts, eggs, tofu, cheese, and peanut butter. Beef, fish, pork, and chicken are also good sources.

The following nutritional information is not always on a food label. A nutrition facts label may include:

Calcium: Calcium keeps the bones strong, helps nerve conduction, promotes strong heart pumping action, and assists with blood clotting. *You are never too young to start taking calcium for bone strength and never too old to stop.* If you have started to develop osteoarthritis, calcium supplements may slow its progression! If you are older than fifty, you should consume one thousand two hundred milligrams of calcium per day.

On the nutrition facts label, calcium will be listed as percentage of daily-recommended amount. For example, Calcium ten percent means that one serving will give you ten percent of your daily-recommended allowance.

Good sources of calcium include: milk, cheese, yogurt, tofu, collards, and sardines. You can buy calcium-fortified foods, which means the food manufacture has added calcium supplements into the food. Good calcium fortified foods are cereal and orange juice.

Take calcium supplements at bedtime. Calcium citrate is a better choice for people over fifty because it absorbs faster in the stomach. Your body needs vitamin D to absorb calcium. Look for calcium supplements that also contain vitamin D supplements.

Iron: Iron carries oxygen in your blood, helps your body to make protein, and changes beta-carotene into vitamin A. Low amounts of iron can cause fatigue, muscle weakness, and headaches. The recommended daily amount of iron, for people fifty to seventy years old, is eight milligrams.

Good iron sources include: red meats, liver, shellfish, poultry, dried beans, dried fruits, and some fortified cereals. Coffee and tea can block the absorption of iron so take your iron supplements with water.

Zinc: Zinc helps your body fight infections and repairs injured body tissues. Your daily zinc intake should be about eight milligrams. Good zinc sources include: meat, fish, poultry, and milk products.

Vitamins

Your body needs vitamins to remain healthy. If you eat properly, you will get most of your vitamin needs met naturally. *Supplements can be beneficial, but they should not be used as an excuse to avoid eating certain food groups!* A daily vitamin that helps you to meet one hundred percent of the recommended daily allowances is safe and encouraged by most health care professionals. Speak to a health care professional before bulking up or following the vitamin craze. Over use of vitamins can cause health problems.

Vitamins are listed as percentages on food labels. *The longer vegetables are cooked the more nutrients they will lose!* Eat vegetables raw or al dente. Here are some basic facts about vitamins:

- **Vitamin A** (Retinol) keeps the skin and mucous membranes healthy, strengthens bones and teeth, and improves night vision. Retinol also keeps the cell walls strong, which helps to fight infections. Good sources of retinol include: vegetables and fruits that are deep green, yellow, or orange. Eggs, milk, cheese, butter, and liver are also good sources. Retinol is a fat-soluble vitamin. This means the unused portions are stored in your body's liver and fat tissue. Excessive amounts can lead to severe fatigue, weakness, blurred vision, joint pain, and even hair loss! Your target intake should be five thousand international units or seven hundred micrograms per day.

- **Vitamin B1** (Thiamin) helps your heart, nerves, and brain to function. Good sources of thiamin include: beef, pork, liver, peas, and whole grain cereals.

- **Vitamin B2** (Riboflavin) helps with the formation of blood cells, keeps your skin healthy, and gives you energy. If you do not get enough riboflavin, your skin becomes dry and your eyes may become very sensitive to light. Good sources of riboflavin include: eggs, milk, cheese, meat, and green leafy vegetables.

- **Vitamin B3** (Niacin) helps your nerves to function, promotes digestion, and keeps your skin healthy. Good sources of niacin include: eggs, nuts, fish, meat, poultry, liver, and brown rice.

- **Vitamin B6** (Pyridoxine) helps to form red blood cells, utilizes protein, and maintains normal brain functioning. Good sources of pyridoxine include: pork, meat, potatoes, mangos, bananas and whole grain cereals.

- **Vitamin B12** (Cobalamin) helps the nerves and brain to function. It also helps your body make DNA. DNA is our genetic fingerprint. Deficiencies in vitamin cobalamin and pyridoxine may be linked to memory loss. Good sources of cobalamin include: eggs, fish, meat, liver, poultry, and milk products.

- **Folic acid** (Folate) helps your body's cells reproduce. It is essential that pregnant women eat large amounts of folate. It may also help to prevent colon cancer and reduce the risk of heart disease. Good sources of folate include: liver, spinach, broccoli, asparagus, kidney beans, and lima beans.

- **Vitamin C** (Ascorbic acid) helps your immune system, promotes healing, and helps to absorb iron. It may reduce your chances of getting certain cancers because it works as an antioxidant. Good sources of ascorbic acid include: fresh fruits (guava, papaya, oranges, grapefruit) and vegetables (especially broccoli). Adults need about seventy-five milligrams per day.

- **Vitamin D** helps to absorb calcium and strengthens bones and teeth. Vitamin D is unique because your body can make its own supply from sunlight! Besides sunlight, good sources of vitamin D include: tuna, salmon, egg yolks, and fortified milk. Vitamin D is a fat-soluble vitamin. Extra vitamin D is stored in the heart, kidney, and blood vessels. This can cause high blood pressure, headaches, loss of appetite, and diarrhea. Adults need about four hundred international units per day or ten micrograms. If you are over seventy, your target intake should be about six hundred international units or fifteen micrograms.

- **Vitamin E** helps form red blood cells and works as an antioxidant to help prevent certain cancers and infections. It may lower your risk of heart disease. Good sources of vitamin E include: milk, almonds, grain cereals, peanut butter, and most vegetable oils. Adults need thirty international units or fifteen milligrams per day. Vitamin E can be bought in a liquid form and topically applied to wounds or cuts. It may help heal the tissue and limit scar formation. *Do not apply vitamin E to any wound until it is thoroughly closed and free of infection.* Do not use on surgical incisions unless approved by the surgeon.

- **Vitamin K** helps the blood to clot. It also binds with calcium and makes the bones stronger. Good sources of vitamin K include: kale, broccoli, spinach, cabbage, beef liver, and green tea. If you are taking an anticoagulant medication (blood thinner), you should limit your intake of foods high in vitamin K.

Eating Right

You need to make a conscious decision to eat the right foods every day. *Do not try to make major or radical dietary changes. Start with small changes and work towards your ultimate goal.* If you want to lose weight, take small steps towards that goal. Rapid weight loss is not safe or healthy. Healthy eating requires a sensible long lasting approach. Read these tips and start making healthy food choices.

Tip Exploration

Tip 48. Read food labels. Use food labels to make healthy choices. Try to limit your intake of saturated and trans fats. Watch your sodium and total carbohydrate intake. Tackle one problem at a time. Ask yourself, "What am I most worried about?" "Is it my weight, sodium intake, or cholesterol?" Trying to change every thing at one time can be overwhelming. Start with baby steps.

Tip 49. Make your plate look like a rainbow. A plate with many different colored foods is more likely to be balanced and healthy. Brightly and naturally colored foods are high in vitamins and nutrients. Eat more green! Mix orange, yellow, red, and green peppers together! Eat bright red beets! Eat some fresh blueberries or cook some yellow corn.

Tip 50. Limit your intake of canned foods and processed meats. Eat fresh when possible. Occasionally eating canned soups or meats is fine, but limit their frequency. Canned foods have large amounts of sodium. Plus, they often have lots of preservatives! Yuk!

Tip 51. Use herbs or spices to add flavor to your food. The taste buds ability to effectively work deteriorates as you age. Experiment with new spices and herbs. You will be pleasantly surprised with the results! Try these tips to improve flavor:

- Add fresh cilantro, rosemary, garlic, or thyme to meat dishes.
- Add chives, parsley, or basil to vegetable dishes.
- Add cumin, saffron, or sweet Hungarian paprika to rice or potatoes.
- Add cinnamon, allspice, or nutmeg to casserole dishes.
- Use balsamic or red wine vinegar on your salads.

Write the name of a new herb or spice you are going to try: _____

Monosodium Glutamate (MSG) is a common ingredient found in Chinese food, canned soups and vegetables, and some frozen prepared meals. MSG is made from the fermentation of corn, sugar beets, or sugar cane. You can have an allergic reaction to this ingredient. Signs of allergic reactions include: numbness, headaches, flushing, sweating, rapid heartbeat, facial swelling, and difficulty breathing. If you experience these symptoms, go directly to the hospital. MSG can also raise your blood sugar and sodium levels. Avoid MSG foods by reading food labels and requesting MSG free foods at restaurants.

Tip 52. Try supplemental drinks. Supplemental products can be used to help fill some nutritional gaps. *They are not a substitute to eating regular meals.* They should be used in conjunction with a healthy diet. Dietitians can direct you to the best supplement to meet your needs. For example, if you lost weight due to a medical problem, you need a supplement with more calories. If you have diabetes or kidney failure, you need a supplement that is especially made to help with those conditions. Lactose free supplements are available. Many companies make nutritional supplements. Use a search engine and type in the phrase "medical nutritional supplements." Visit the Ensure's site at www.ensure.com or www.ross.com for numerous recipe ideas. You can cook with it or add it to muffins, soups, or casseroles for added nutritional value!

Tip 53. Eat small and frequent meals. Eating three large meals per day worked when you were younger, but you may find that eating four or five small meals per day makes you feel better. Your digestive system slows as you age, so it is easier for your body to digest smaller portions than big heavy meals. This does not mean snacking on chips in front of the television! Start your morning with cereal and coffee and then in the middle of the morning have some fruit. Eat your sandwich at noon and then in the middle of the afternoon have a piece of fresh fruit or yogurt. Eat your supper. Avoid bedtime snacking.

Tip 54. Get good dental care. Teeth are needed to properly chew food. It is difficult to absorb nutrients from poorly chewed foods. If you have dentures, make sure they fit securely. Poor fitting dentures are of no value to anyone! Visit your dentist on an annual basis. Change your toothbrush frequently.

Tip 55. Drink your milk! Milk may cause a stomach upset because your small intestine has lost its ability to make lactase. Lactase digests (breaks down) the sugar in milk called lactose. Lactose that remains inside your intestines causes nausea, bloating, gas, and diarrhea. Taking lactase enzyme supplements may help alleviate the symptoms. Whole milk products have a higher fat content, which slows the rate of digestion resulting in a gradual release of lactose. Therefore you may find that whole milk is better for you than skim milk. Consider trying lactose free milk or soymilk.

Tip 56. Stop eating two hours before bedtime. Do not lie down on the couch right after eating. Lying down slows your body's digestive process. You will feel more bloated and stuffed.

Tip 57 Use antacids with caution. Occasional attacks of indigestion are normal. If you experience indigestion more than twice a week, on a regular basis, seek medical attention. You may have acid reflux disease. Acid reflux disease can be easily treated with medications and diet.

Tip 58. Explore new food cultures. America is a potpourri of multiple nationalities. New and exciting restaurants have arrived to celebrate these cultural delights. Do not be afraid to try something new. Try Japanese cuisine (and no it is not just raw fish) or try Mexican (and no it is not always spicy). Try a Thai food appetizer. If you are unsure about what to order, ask the waitress or waiter for recommendations. Go for it!

Tip 59. Share casseroles with neighbors or friends. Do you love casseroles, but hate the leftovers? Cook your favorite casserole dish and give some to your neighbor. Your neighbors will be very grateful!

Tip 60. Keep it safe! According to the United States Food and Drug Administration, there are about seventy-six million cases of food borne illnesses every year! Think "safe food preparation." The most common causes of food borne illnesses are viruses, bacteria, and parasites. These things arrive as "uninvited dinner guests." You can quickly escort them out the door! Some safe food preparation tips include:

- Thaw food in the refrigerator and not on the counter.
- Use two different knives: one to cut raw meat and one to cut your vegetables.
- Place doggie bags into the refrigerator as soon as possible and eat them within twenty-four hours.
- Change the dishtowels at least every two days: once per day is best.
- Change sponges at least once a month. Sponges grow bacteria.
- Date frozen foods and throw them away if not used within a few months.

- Use meat thermometers when cooking.

- Refrigerate leftovers within two hours of cooking and dispose of them if not eaten within three days.

- Do not use cans with dents or bulges.

- Remove cooked stuffing from turkeys or chickens before putting them into the refrigerator.

- Keep non-food items (paper and mail) off the counter when preparing foods.

- Keep your refrigerator at 40° Fahrenheit and your freezer at 0° Fahrenheit.

Tip 61. Be a savvy food shopper. "Last sell date," means the last day that the item can be sold, no exceptions! "Best if used by date," means in order to get the best flavor and nutrients from this item it has to be eaten by this date. Make a shopping list before going to the store. Stick to it! Avoid the end of aisle specials because they often are snack food traps! Most stores place the healthier foods on the perimeter aisles; stay out of the middle aisles where snacks foods are nestled. *Become a perimeter shopper!*

Tip 62. Make eating fun. Use nice place settings. Light the candles even when eating alone. Eat outside. Avoid eating in the living room with the television on; it is a bad habit. Add texture to your dinner plate. *Crunchy foods will liven up your meal!* Go to the senior center for an occasional meal.

Tip 63. Allow yourself a treat. Fulfill your cravings. If you love ice cream, enjoy a bowl. If you love chocolate, eat a piece. Completely barring cravings will result in a rebound of overindulgence. *Indulge not overindulge!*

Tip 64. Conserve energy by using ramekins. Preparing meals is tiring. If you get tired preparing meals, try these suggestions:

- Cook in stages.

- Put cut vegetables into ramekin dishes and cook them later.

- Put cut potatoes into cold water and cook them later.

- Use paper plates and plastic utensils to make clean up easier.

- Make one large casserole dish and freeze it in small individual containers.

Eating takes energy. Spread out the process. Save your energy for eating.

Internet Resources

- Go to the American Heart Association (www.americanheart.org) web site for healthy eating information.

- Go to American Diabetes Association (www.diabetes.org) web site for diet guidelines for people with Diabetes.

- Go to the Food and Drug Administration (www.fda.gov) web site for information on food borne illnesses and safe food preparation. Visit their other site www.foodsafety.gov and get your "Bad Bug Book!"

- Go to the American Dietetic Association (www.eatright.org) web site for some helpful information regarding nutrition and healthy eating.

- Go to the Food Allergy and Anaphylaxis Network (www.foodallergy.org) web site for helpful information on living with food allergies.

- Go to the Food TV (www.foodtv.com) web site for new recipes and cooking tips.

- Go to a search engine and type these words: food safety, nutrition, and healthy diet.

5

Digestion and Elimination:
"What is constipation?"
"What is an overactive bladder?"

Just the Facts

Food goes from the mouth to your esophagus and then to the stomach. The stomach begins the process of breaking food down into small parts. These small parts leave the stomach and go into the small intestine. After the small intestine, it travels through the large intestine and finally reaches the rectum. Most nutrients are absorbed in the small intestine. Left over materials are either stored as fat or eliminated. Your body eliminates waste through either urine or feces. Feces are commonly referred to as bowel movements. No one enjoys talking about these issues, but it is necessary. You can not live without a strong system that digests food and eliminates waste.

There are many digestive system illnesses. Unlike heart problems, these illnesses generally are not life threatening. However, they can lead to serious problems if not properly treated. Three common digestive system illnesses are digestive ulcers, urinary incontinence, and constipation.

Digestive Ulcers

About five hundred thousand new cases of digestive ulcers are diagnosed every year and about four million people will experience a recurrent problem. A digestive ulcer is the erosion of the mucous membrane. Digestive ulcers can be in the stomach, esophagus, or small intestine.

What causes ulcers? The three major causes include:

- Medications.

- Infections.

- Acid over secretion disorders.

Non-steroidal anti-inflammatory (NSAID) medications are common culprits. These medications are used to treat illnesses including: arthritis, headaches, sore muscles, menstrual cramps, and aches and pains. Examples of these medications include: aspirin, ibuprofen (Advil, Motrin), Vioxx and Naproxen. Digestive ulcers develop from the accumulative long term use of these medications. *Using these medications periodically will probably not result in an ulcer formation.*

The helicobacter pylorus is a normal bacterium that lives in the membranes of your intestines. It can overgrow and can cause an ulcer to form. This bacterium is the cause of about ninety-five percent of all digestive ulcers. There are only a few disorders that can cause acid over secretion.

If you have a stomach ulcer, you may experience:

- Indigestion.

- Heartburn.

- Weight loss.

- A dull ache in the stomach area.

- Being awoken at night from the pain.

If you have a duodenum (part of small intestine) ulcer, you may experience:

- Heartburn.

- Stomach pains relieved with eating or antacids.

- Weight gain.

- Discomfort that is felt two to four hours after a meal.

- Discomfort that feels worse after taking aspirin, drinking coffee, or drinking citrus juices.

Hemorrhage and perforation are the most serious ulcer complications. Hemorrhage means that the ulcer site begins bleeding. You start vomiting bright red blood or you may notice your stools turning black. Perforation means that the ulcer has created a hole through the stomach wall and its contents are going into your abdomen. Severe pain will be the primary symptom. Go to your local emergency room for an evaluation.

Indigestion is a symptom of a problem. The common signs of indigestion include: nausea, heartburn, bloated feeling, discomfort in the upper abdomen after eating, which is often relieved by belching. Tell your doctor how often you experience indigestion. He will be able to determine its cause. A sensation of indigestion may also be a sign of a heart attack. If your indigestion feeling does not promptly resolve, seek medical attention.

Urinary Incontinence

Thirteen million Americans have some form of a urinary incontinence problem. It bothers about one in every ten women. Less than half of all people with this disorder seek medical attention. Why? Do not hide in the closet. Leaking urine with a sneeze or a cough is *not* a normal part of aging. Medical treatments can help you. Talk to your doctor. Be honest. Approximately eighteen billion dollars a year is spent on urinary incontinence treatments (medications, pads, and surgical procedures). Most cases of urinary incontinence can easily be treated with exercises or medications. Surgery is generally not needed.

There are five major types of urinary incontinence problems. They include:

- Overflow incontinence: A blockage in either the bladder or the urethra (tube that takes urine from the bladder to the outside) causing the urine to be involuntarily released.

- Stress incontinence: Urethra muscle weakness causes urine to be released with coughing, sneezing, or laughing.

- Urge incontinence: A sudden urge to urinate is felt, but you can not control it. The urine is involuntarily released.

- Functional incontinence: Complete urinating control is present, but you are unable to reach the bathroom because of other problems (arthritis, pain).

- Reflex incontinence: A total loss of urinating control is present and due to a neurological problem.

What else causes urinary incontinence? Some of the most common causes include: obesity, menopause, enlarged prostate, hysterectomies, and obstructions from tumors, growths or scar tissue. Smoking and excessive caffeine ingestion may also contribute to this problem.

Certain medications can cause these problems. For example, Artane (Trihexane) a Parkinson medication can cause urinary problems. Talk to your pharmacist and have all your medications reviewed for potential urinary side effects. If you are taking medications that can cause urinary problems and you are experiencing problems, talk to your doctor. Do not stop the medications without consulting your doctor first.

Doctors can diagnosis urinary incontinence problems by taking an accurate medical history. Ultrasounds, urine tests, and blood tests may also be needed.

The risks for not treating this condition include: anxiety, depression, urinary tract infections, and some skin problems. Urine has acidic properties. If urine remains on the skin, you may develop skin infections, rashes, and ulcers.

Constipation

You do *not* need to have a daily bowel movement! Some people have a bowel movement every two or three days. If you had a bowel movement every other day when you were forty, do not expect to have one every day now that you are sixty!

Constipation is medically defined as the inability to have a bowel movement or having recurrent movements that are hard and difficult to pass. Waste products move through the colon by an action called peristalsis. Peristalsis slows down because of various reasons. As you age, the colon becomes more stretched and less elastic. This makes it difficult for bowel movements to move through easily.

Medications can cause constipation. Pain medications are the number one offender, especially narcotics. Other medications include: aspirin, antihistamines, some heart medications, aluminum salts in acids, iron supplements, and certain antidepressants.

Your colon functions best when you are active. A couch potato lifestyle is not good for promoting regular bowel activity. A daily walk will keep the colon happy and your heart!

About ninety-four thousand cases of colon cancer are discovered every year. It is the second most common cancer site. Colon cancer kills approximately fifty thousand people every year, but it is one of the most treatable forms of cancer. *Early detection is key*. No one ever said a colonoscopy was fun, but it can save your life. Do not listen to the stories your friends have told you about the procedure. Medications are always given during the procedure to help you relax. If cancer is found, surgery is the primary treatment. Radiation or chemotherapy may also be needed.

Solving These Problems

These topics do not make great dinner conversation, but they are appropriate concerns and should be discussed with your doctor. Remember, tip number one, get a good doctor. You need to feel comfortable enough with your doctor to discuss these issues. Do not feel embarrassed talking to your doctor. They want to help you feel better. Do not rely on your neighbor's home remedies. Some home remedies may work, but others can land you in the hospital! Here are some tips to help you with the common digestive system illnesses.

Tip Exploration

Tip 65. Try non-medication treatments for digestive ulcers. Stop smoking. Smoking is not only bad for your heart and lungs, but it increases stomach acid production. Avoid coffee and tea. Limit soda intake, especially ones with caffeine. Avoid aspirin and other NSAID medications.

In severe cases, doctors can perform various surgeries to treat ulcers. A vagotomy cuts the vagus nerve resulting in acid secretion reduction. An antrectomy is the removal of part of the stomach. Surgery is rarely needed.

Tip 66. Talk to your doctor about medication options for digestive ulcers. These medications protect the stomach and mucous membranes from damage. If the ulcer is caused by the helicobacter pylori bacterium, a combination of medications will be ordered. The combination includes:

- Antibiotics (tetracycline, metronidazole) to get rid of the bacteria.

- H2 blockers (cimetidine, ranitidine) to help block histamines that stimulate acid secretion.

- Proton pump inhibitors (omeprazole, lansoprazole) to stop the pumping action of acid into the stomach.

- Stomach lining protectors ((bismuth preparation) to coat the stomach walls.

If you are taking NSAIDs and are at risk for developing stomach ulcers, Cytotec can be prescribed to help prevent ulcers from developing. Diarrhea is a common side effect to this medication, but it is usually self-controlling.

Tip 67. Try Kegel exercises for urinary incontinence problems. Kegel exercises will strengthen the pelvic floor muscles. These exercises help control urinary stress incontinence problems. Contract your pelvic floor muscles for ten seconds and then release the muscles. Repeat ten times. Do this exercise at least once per day; twice per day is preferable. Try this exercise now. You will need to do these exercises for at least six weeks to strengthen the muscles. *Never do Kegel exercises while urinating*. This will stop the urine flow and can lead to urinary tract infections or other problems.

Tip 68. Try bladder training exercises. These exercises treat urge incontinence problems. Basically you place yourself on a toileting schedule. Plan to go to the bathroom at eight o'clock, ten o'clock, noon, and so on, even if you do not feel the urge to urinate. You may need to start with smaller time intervals depending on your condition. Increase the time intervals until an acceptable time frame has been reached. Avoid drinking water or other fluids after six o'clock in the evening.

If bladder training is not effective, consider using absorbent pads. These pads help to keep the urine away from sensitive skin and prevent embarrassing leaks. Men can be fitted with a condom like device that has a plastic tube attached to drain the urine. In severe cases, men and women can have catheters directly inserted into the bladder. Catheters have complications and should *only* be used after all other options have been tried.

Tip 69. Talk to your doctor about pelvic floor treatments. Three common pelvic floor treatments include: electrical stimulation, vaginal weight training, and pessary insertion. Electrical stimulation is a painless procedure in which a probe causes the muscles to contract and thus they get stronger. This stimulation works for people with stress and urge incontinence problems. Vaginal weight training promotes muscle strength. A pessary is a stiff ring inserted into the vagina that helps to reposition the urethra. This works for stress incontinence problems. The pessary is inserted in a doctor's office.

Tip 70. Talk to your doctor about medication options for urinary incontinence. Detrol is a medication used to treat an overactive bladder. Dry mouth and headaches are the most common side effects. Avoid driving or other potentially hazardous activity for the first few days as a precaution from any visual effects related to the drug. Abnormal visual effects are temporary and resolve when the medication is stopped. Other medication options include: collagen injections, estrogen hormone replacements, anticholinergics, and antispasmodics.

Tip 71. Treat constipation with good eating habits. Eat fresh fruits and consume plenty of fiber. A sudden increase in fiber can cause gas and bloating. Fiber supplements take about forty-eight hours to begin working.

Tip 72. Use laxative medications with caution. Laxatives are *not* intended for daily consumption. Thoroughly shake any laxative solutions before taking them. Drink a large glass of water with all laxative medications. If you have diabetes, check the label for sugar and use a sugar free psyllium brand.

Tip 73. Do not strain when having a bowel movement. Straining with a bowel movement is very dangerous. It causes stress on your heart and contributes to hemorrhoid development. Sit straight on the toilet. Maintain good posture. If your feet do not touch the floor, use a footstool. This helps to relax your back muscles and can make defecation easier.

Stool softeners help to decrease the need to strain. Docusate sodium (colace or duosol) works by increasing the amount of liquid absorbed into the stool making it easier to pass. It should *not* be used to treat constipation, but prevent it from forming. It takes one to three days before you will notice a difference. Use it occasionally unless otherwise directed by your doctor.

Tip 74. Stop diarrhea as soon as possible. Diarrhea can lead to life threatening dehydration because of the loss of electrolytes and water. Treat diarrhea with the BRAT diet. The BRAT diet includes:

- Bananas.

- Rice.

- Applesauce.

- Toast or tapioca.

Applesauce and bananas contain pectin that helps to absorb extra water. Avoid fresh fruits and hot drinks. Try various over the counter medications to treat diarrhea. Follow the bottles instructions for maximum dosage. Do not exceed the limit. If you develop abdominal pain or the diarrhea lasts for more than three days, seek medical attention.

Tip 75. Try these tips to control gas problems. Air that enters the intestinal tract has to be eliminated. The trick is to prevent excessive air from entering the system. If you have breathing problems (asthma, heart failure), you are more likely to use your mouth to breathe. Mouth breathers have more gas. Learn the proper way to use your inhalers. Tightly seal your lips around the mouthpiece.

Use a spacer on your inhaler. Ask the pharmacist for a pamphlet showing you the proper way to use a spacer and inhaler. There is a right way and wrong way!

Gas also enters the tract when using straws, sucking hard candies, and chewing gum. Foods can contribute to gas formation. Examples of gas forming foods include: peas, beans, cabbage, broccoli, cauliflower, and brussell sprouts.

Activity, such as walking, can help alleviate gas discomfort. Try to stay erect for at least thirty minutes after eating. Lying on the couch will increase gas discomfort.

Internet Resources

- Go to the Simon Foundation for Continence (www. simonfoundation.org) web site for suggestions and resources for people suffering from urinary incontinence problems.

- Go to the National Digestive Diseases Information Clearinghouse (www.digestive.niddk.nih.gov) web site for information on various stomach, intestinal, and kidney disorders.

- Go to the American Foundation for Urologic Diseases (www.afud.org) web site for resource information about various kidney and urinary diseases.

- Go to the National Association for Continence (www.nafc.org) web site for information about preventing, diagnosing, and treating incontinence problems.

- Go to the American Cancer Society (www.cancer.org) for more information on preventing, diagnosing, and treating colon cancer.

- Go to a search engine and type these words: constipation, incontinence, colon cancer, and digestive ulcers.

6

Exercise: "Why should I exercise?"
"How do I start?"

Just the Facts

What is exercise? You have heard that term over and over again, but do you really know what it means? *Exercise is a physical or mental activity that follows a repetitive pattern with the goal of improving or maintaining fitness.* Physical activity alone does *not* constitute exercise. Physical activity can help you burn calories, but it will not help to tone or strengthen your body unless it follows a repetitive plan. Most people are physically active. You get up in the morning, get out of bed, walk to the bath room, shower, make lunches, take out the trash, and fold the clothes. These activities all require physical activity, but they do not serve as exercise. You must exercise your mind and your body.

The phrase "no pain means no gain" is not accurate. Exercise should *not* be painful or lead to discomfort. If it does, you have over done it. Muscle pain following exercise is due to poor stretching or an overzealous approach. *Use the ten percent rule.* Increase the exercise duration and intensity by ten percent each week until you reach your maximum level.

Exercise can become an "exercise in frustration." Do not let that happen. Make your exercise routine fun and enjoyable. If you become frustrated, you will not continue doing it!

"I have never exercised before so why should I start now?" There are numerous health benefits to exercising. Exercise helps your heart, lungs, stomach, digestive tract, and even your brain. It helps with medical conditions including: arthritis, diabetes, osteoporosis, heart disease, and high blood pressure. Doing good breathing exercises will help your lungs. You will sleep better at night after getting some exercise. Socialization is also a benefit of regular exercising.

Exercise Excuses

The news is filled with stories about the benefits to exercising, but nine of ten Americans do not exercise on a regular basis. Why? The common reasons for not exercising include: too busy, too tired, too sick, can not afford to join a gym, or do not know where to start. Which excuse is yours? Here is an answer to your excuse.

Too busy? The American Heart Association recommends thirty minutes per day three times per week. That is only ninety minutes per week! How many minutes per day do you watch television? How many minutes per day do you sit and read? How many minutes per day do you lie in bed thinking about what you want to do? Most people can find thirty minutes per day to do some form of exercise. If you can not find thirty free minutes, try fifteen.

Too tired? Exercising will actually invigorate you. You will feel energized and excited to try new things after getting some exercise. If you physically feel too tired to exercise, you need to talk to your doctor about a medically approved exercise plan. For example, he may recommend a cardiac rehabilitation program that is designed to help people with heart disease become stronger. There are other types of medically approved exercise programs.

Too Sick? Only a few medical conditions warrant a *complete* stoppage of exercise. Ask you doctor if you have any medical condition that does *not* allow you to exercise. Many illnesses can cause pain and discomfort making exercising an uncomfortable event, but it is important to get some exercise every day. You need to keep your body and joints moving. In the next chapter, you will learn about physical and occupational therapists. These professionals can teach you or your caregiver how to perform certain range of motion exercises. A range of motion exercise is a specific exercise program that puts a joint through all its natural movements. Joints that are not used will become stiff and can permanently lose their ability to work. You do not want that to happen!

Can not afford to join a gym? You do not need to belong to a gym or health club. There are numerous ways you can exercise in your house without expensive equipment. Start by buying an exercise videotape or compact disc. Look for special senior citizens ones!

I do not know where to start. This is the easiest excuse to fix. Just start small. Doing something is better than doing nothing! *The most dangerous part of an exercise program is not enrolling in one!* Get moving!

Types of Physical Exercise

Jogging and skiing are great ways to exercise, but do not attempt these exercises if you are not in good physical shape. Here are three exercise programs that will help you get into shape!

- Yoga is a five thousand year old discipline that combines breathing, meditation, and posture routines. The goal is to promote good balance and strength. Yoga's breathing exercises teaches you to regulate your inhalation and exhalation time using pranayama. Pranayama means you inhale and exhale slowly, deeply, and at a constant rate. Posture exercises help your bones, muscles, and nervous system.

- Joseph Pilates was born in Germany and suffered from asthma and rheumatic fever. He created an exercise program to tackle his health problems. The program was later named after him and has become very popular in the past ten years. Pilates consists of balance, strength, and flexibility training. It aims to decrease stress and promote lean muscles without the "bulking" up look. It focuses on the *quality* of the muscle exercises versus the *quantity* of the exercises.

- Tai Chi is a type of martial arts program that enhances balance and body strengthening through slow, graceful, and precision body movements. The National Institute on Health (www.nih.gov) and the National Institute on Aging (www.nia.gov) recommend this type of exercise program for older people. *Recent studies have shown that participants in Tai Chi programs have significantly less falls than non-program participants.*

Home videos can be purchased for these exercise programs, but it is recommended that beginners take an initial lesson with a professional trainer. This person will teach you how to safely and correctly do the exercises.

If you develop chest pain or tightness in your chest, stop exercising. If you experience a fluttering sensation in your chest, stop exercising. It is normal to have some shortness of breath while exercising, but you should *never* feel like you can not catch your breath. Stop exercising if you become dizzy or lightheaded. If you experience any of these symptoms, sit down and rest for a few minutes. If the symptoms do not go away within a few minutes, call your local emergency services number.

Just Get Moving

You are now ready to start exercising. There are fourteen exercise tips in this section. Do not attempt to do all fourteen in one day. Start by selecting two or three exercises and add a few more each week.

Tip Exploration

Tip 76. Set goals. It is human nature to procrastinate. If you do not write down a few goals, you will never start or continue an exercise program. *A goal must be reasonable and obtainable.* A good exercise goal includes mental, physical, and social activities. For example, "I will do two mental activities per day, fifteen minutes of physical activities per day, and attend one social activity per week." This goal is reasonable, achievable, and makes logical sense. An unreasonable goal for most people would be to, "I will run ten miles every day, do twelve crossword puzzles, and attend six social functions per week."

Get a pen and finish this sentence: I will do _____ mental activities per week, _____ minutes of physical activity per week, and attend _____ social functions per week.

Tip 77. Plan your reward. Rewards allow us to celebrate accomplishments. They serve as motivators. *Give yourself a reward for meeting your goals.* You can not count on anyone else to reward you. You need to take charge of your own destiny. A reward is something small that will make you feel special. It may be an ice cream cone, bouquet of flowers, or tickets to a movie.

Finish this sentence: If I meet my goals for this week, I will give myself a

_____.

Tip 78. Get a partner. If you have a partner, you are more likely to achieve your goals. A partner can encourage and motivate you to reach your goal. Your partner could be your neighbor, your kids, or someone who lives a thousand miles away. It would be nice to have a partner to exercise with, but get on the phone and call someone. Encourage them to read this book and start exercising. As the saying goes, "two heads are better than one!"

Write down the name of your partner. _____

Tip 79. Plan your mental exercises. You are probably thinking, "I use my brain every day. It does not need any special exercises." Not true! Your brain tissue is a very specialized organ. For example, reading uses one part of your brain, solving crossword puzzles uses a different part, playing scrabble uses yet another part.

Think about what you normally do and find something new to try. Examples of mental exercises include:

- Crossword puzzles or word searches.
- Board games such as Scrabble, Monopoly or Battleship. Why should kids have all the fun playing these board games?
- Jigsaw puzzles.
- Three dimensional jigsaw puzzles.
- Chess, checkers, cribbage, or backgammon.
- Hand held video games.
- Computer games.

Write down three new mental exercises you are going to try: _____
_____

Give yourself a deadline for trying those exercises: _____

Tip 80. Plan your social activities. What about going to the movies? Go out to lunch or dinner. Visit an old friend. Have you been to a museum lately? Maybe a basketball, baseball, or football game would be interesting. The objective is to find some activity that causes you to get out of the house and talk to new people.

Write down three social activities that you will do this month: _____
_____

Tip 81. Volunteer for an organization. There are numerous opportunities to give back to your community. Consider volunteering for:

- Schools.
- Libraries.
- Hospitals.
- Nursing homes.
- Senior centers.
- Humane society offices.
- Literacy programs.
- American Red Cross. Volunteers are always needed at blood drives.

Write down a place that you would like to volunteer: _____
Get their phone number and write it down here: _____

Tip 82. Plan your physical exercises. These exercises are good starting points. They will help you to stretch and move your body. *Never* do anything that causes pain or undue stress. Start slow. Try five repetitions and then progress to ten or fifteen.

1. Lie flat on your back in bed. Place your arms at your side. Lift one leg a few inches off the bed. Hold it for a count of ten. Repeat five times. Repeat with your other leg. If you have back or hip problems, do not do this exercise.

2. Lie flat on your back in bed. Pretend your arms and legs are wings. Spread your wings (arms and legs) out as far as you can. Bring your arms and legs back. Repeat ten times. Try to keep your arms and legs as straight as possible.

3. Sit in a chair without a table in front of you. Keep your shoulders back and chest out. Keep your feet flat on the floor. Bring your arms straight out in front of you and raise them into the air as high as you can. Hold your arms up for the count of ten and then bring your arms back to your sides. Repeat five times. Next, straighten one leg and raise it into the air. Hold it for a count of ten. Do five repetitions. Repeat with your other leg.

4. Sit at a table with your arms resting on the table. Grab a can of soup with one hand and lift it into the air. Hold your arm straight up in the air for a count of ten. Put your arm down. Repeat this five times. Repeat with your other arm. Canned tomatoes can be exchanged for cans of soup, as you get stronger. Gradually work up to a gallon of water!

5. Sit at a table with your arms relaxed. Place a pencil under the tips of your fingers and roll the pencil out until your arm is straight. Roll your arm back and forth ten times. Repeat with your other arm.

6. Sit at a table with your arms relaxed. Grab a pencil in your hand and make a tight fist. Hold it tight for a count of ten. Relax your fist. Do five repetitions. Repeat with your other hand.

7. While watching television, do ten shoulder shrugs. Then, straighten your arms and do ten circle motions. Watch television in a recliner. Recliners require strength and force to sit up. Do not watch television in bed. It is a bad habit. Get the television out of the bedroom!

8. Rock in a rocking chair. Start with your feet flat on the floor and then push off with your feet. Pull yourself back using your upper body muscles. Repeat ten times.

9. Take a towel and pretend you are drying your back. Hold one corner of the towel over your right shoulder and grab the other end of the towel at left hip. Pull the towel with your left arm and then again with your right hand. Do five towel pulls. Switch the towel to the other side and repeat. If you have shoulder problems, do not do this exercise.

10. Get a rubber band and put your thumb and index finger in it. Stretch your index finger out as far as the rubber band will allow. Do five stretches. Move the rubber band to your middle finger and repeat. The purpose of this exercise is to move and stretch all ten fingers. This exercise also helps the muscles in your hand. If you have a history of carpal tunnel or any other hand problems, do not do this exercise.

11. Grab a tennis ball with your hand and squeeze tightly. Hold the squeeze for the count of ten. Relax and repeat five times. Switch hands and repeat. If you have a history of carpal tunnel or any other hand problems, do not do this exercise.

Take your pencil and circle three exercises that you are going to try. Come back next week and circle three more. Continue until you have tried all the exercises!

Tip 83. Get a pedometer. Walking is a great way to exercise. It improves your balance, endurance, and circulation. It helps to control your blood pressure and lowers your cholesterol. You can buy pedometers in department or sport equipment stores. Wear the pedometer for one week. Keep track of your daily mileage. Set a goal of increasing your walking mileage by five or ten percent each week. Start by taking leisurely strolls, advance to brisk walks, and progress to power walking.

Where is the closest store that sells pedometers? _____

Finish this sentence: I will buy a pedometer by _____ (date).

Indoor shopping malls are great places for walking. They are safe, well lit, and have smooth walking surfaces. Avoid walking on roads with curves or hills especially during dawn or sunset hours. Do not carry your wallet or money with you while walking. You can increase your walking distances by simply parking your car in farthest parking spot from the stores entrance!

Tip 84. Have a good laugh! Laughter is actually good exercise for your lungs. A good laugh helps you inhale and exhale deeply. This action helps your lung tissues get enough oxygen. It also makes your lungs stronger and better at loosening phlegm. Loose phlegm is easier for your lungs to cough out!

Tip 85. Buy good exercise equipment. Use extreme caution when buying used sports equipment because parts may be loose or missing. If you buy a bike or any other equipment at a tag sale, get it checked for stability and safety. You can use milk jugs filled with water instead of buying expensive weights. Change the water to sand to make them even heavier!

Tip 86. Form a telephone call tree system with your friends. A tree call system is a preplanned daily calling program organized by a group of friends. The purpose of the system is to form a safety net for older people who live alone. This is how the system works: Sue calls Brenda at nine, Brenda then calls Marie at ten, Marie calls Marge at eleven and so on until everyone on the list has been called. The last person calls the first caller to complete the circle. If someone does not answer the telephone, additional measures are taken to make sure everything is fine. Many senior centers are creating tree call systems. You can easily start one!

Tip 87. Return to school. Call your local community college for a brochure. Most community colleges offer credit and non-credit courses. Take credit courses and get your degree. Fulfill your dream. Take non-credit courses, such as, cooking, gardening, photography, or painting. You will be meet new people and acquire a new talent.

Tip 88. Get a pet. A dog is a great companion and mood elevator. If you do not want a full time dog, offer to dog sit your neighbor's dog for a few days. Cats, fish, birds, and hamsters also make good pets.

Tip 89. Turn on the music! Music is a motivator. It gets you moving. Turn off the television, turn off the news, and turn on your favorite musical group. Play music while cleaning.

Tip 90. Stop every fifteen minutes and drink a glass of water while exercising. Water replacement is essential when exercising. Avoid alcoholic beverages, soda, or other caffeine beverages.

Internet Resources

- Go to the Humane Society (<u>www.hsus.org</u>) web site for information on adopting a pet. Call your local chapter for volunteer opportunities.

- Go to the American Red Cross (<u>www.redcross.org</u>) web site for information on various volunteer opportunities.

- Go to National Senior Games Association (<u>www.nationalseniorgames.org</u>) web site for information on the Senior Olympics. Go for it! Get that gold medal!

- Go to a search engine and type in these words: senior exercising, yoga, pilates, and tai chi.

7

Help! "Who can help me?"
"What devices can help me?"

Just the Facts

There are people and resources available to help you. Reach out and grab them! Ask for help. Do not be shy or embarrassed to ask for assistance. These services may be covered by your health care insurance.

Who can help me? There are six medical professionals that can help you at home. Each one is unique and provides a different service. Here is a closer at these professionals.

- *Physical therapist:* This medical professional can improve your strength, mobility, and gait. Gait refers to your ability to walk and balance yourself. These therapists can perform various treatments including: exercise, massage, water therapies, and whirlpools. Physical therapists can help people with various lung problems. They can perform activities to loosen chest congestion and help to get that "stuff" out of the lungs.

- *Occupational therapist:* An occupational therapist focuses on improving your upper body strength. They can teach you new ways to perform activities of daily living using modifications based on your needs. "Activities of daily living" is a common medical phrase that refers to any task that you need to perform on a regular basis to live. For example, cooking, cleaning, bathing, and shopping are all activities of daily living. The therapist will teach you new ways to do these tasks or will fit you with adaptive devices to help you do the tasks. For example, assume your arthritis does not allow you to open jars. The therapist will teach you how to use an adaptive device to open jars. If one arm is weak and makes cooking dinner difficult, the therapist will teach you new ways to cook dinner compensating for that weak arm.

- *Speech pathologist*: This medical professional can improve your ability to communicate. They help with speech, hearing, and swallowing problems. If someone you know has had a stroke and has difficulty communicating, ask the doctor for a referral to a speech pathologist. Trouble communicating can be very frustrating for you, your family members, and friends. Give a speech pathologist an opportunity to help you. It is well worth your time!

- *Social worker*: This medical professional is like the ringmaster! They direct you or other medical professionals in the right direction. They can provide you with information about local resources and can help you complete financial or legal forms. If a loved needs nursing home placement, ask the doctor for a social worker referral to help you with this process. They will help you with the paperwork. Most nursing homes have waiting lists for openings. A social worker can help you get your name onto a waiting list.

- *Registered nurse:* Nurses can do many things including: organizing your medications, acting as a liaison with doctors, providing education, and performing various treatments. They can teach you information about your diseases including: causes, signs and symptoms, diagnostic procedures, and treatment options. You can hire home care nurses through visiting nurse associations or privately. The majority of private duty nurses provide excellent care. If you decide to hire private duty nurses, ask a minimum of three references and verify their licensure through your states department of public health.

- *Home health aide:* They can help with bathing, exercising, and perform basic treatments (dressing changes). *Each state has specific laws that govern their level of practice.* Home health aides usually work under the direction of nurses. It is possible to hire private duty aides. If you decide to hire private duty aides, ask for a minimum of three references and hire graduates from certified nursing assistant programs or other state approved programs.

There are two other groups of people that can help you. These people are *not* medically trained. They include:

- *Homemakers*: Homemakers can help you with certain housekeeping chores. They can help with cooking, cleaning, shopping, and laundry. Always ask for references before hiring private homemakers. Some insurance plans will pay for their services.

- *Companions:* Companions can assist you with various jobs or errands. Most companions are hired to provide company to homebound people. For example, assume your spouse has Alzheimer's disease. It may be difficult for you to leave the house and do some personal errands. A companion will sit with your spouse while you do these errands. Most insurance companies will *not* pay for this service, but your mental health and well being may outweigh the expense. Look in the phone book and compare prices. Getting away for one or two hours per week can rejuvenate your soul. Take care of yourself first or you will not be able to care for your spouse!

Devices

What devices can help me? A device is available to help you with every possible need. You can purchase these items in pharmacies, medical supply stores, or on the Internet. Ask the sales representative or the clerical staff in your doctor's office if your health insurance will reimburse all or part of the cost. Reimbursement depends on the type of item, your medical condition, and your insurance plan.

Tip Exploration

Tip 91. Obtain a referral from your doctor for the above health care professionals. Ask for a referral. Be assertive and say, "I am having trouble with my hands. I think an occupational therapist may be able to help me. Can you refer me to one?" If you timidly say to the doctor, "Can you do anything for me," you will not get the answer that you wanted. It is important to ask for the services that you need. Do not be shy.

Clarify if your insurance will pay for the referral visit. The doctor's clerical staff will be able to answer this question for you.

Tip 92. Do your homework before hiring private duty help. Check at least three references. Ask a family member to be present when interviewing private duty professionals. If they are bonded, ask for proof. *Follow your gut instinct.* If you do not feel comfortable with them, do not hire them. Ask an accountant for recommendations regarding paying for their services and claiming them on your taxes.

Tip 93. Canes provide stability when walking. Canes come in various forms. A simple cane will have one leg, tripod canes will have three legs, and quad canes will have four legs. Tripod and quad canes provide more stability. When using a cane, you should:

- Select the proper size. It should be level with the hipbone and allow your elbow to be flexed comfortably at about a twenty degree angle.

- Hold the cane in the unaffected (stronger) hand and advance it with the affected (weaker) limb. In other words, if your left leg is weak, place the cane in your right hand. Advance the cane when you advance your left leg.

A cane is not made for weight bearing; it is only a supportive device. If you use a cane to keep yourself up, you should switch to a walker.

Does this sound familiar? "Look! I can walk without my cane. I will hold onto the tables instead!" Do not test yourself. Holding or leaning on tables to walk is not safe. Tables can easily tip over. Prevention is the number one goal.

Tip 94. Walkers provide a broader sense of stability when walking. Walkers come in two different forms. A basic walker has four standard legs; a rolling walker has two standard legs and two legs with wheels. The basic walker is the most economical and the best place to start. Rolling walkers are recommended for people that are weaker and have a hard time lifting the walker to ambulate. Walkers are measured the same way as the cane. When walking with a walker, remember these tips:

- Begin by standing straight up with the walker in front of you. It is important to stand up straight and not stoop over.

- Advance the walker ten to twelve inches.

- Then step forward to the walker. Make sure that you lift your legs and feet when walking.

- Keep your head up while walking. Look forward; do not look down.

- Do not shuffle your feet because it increases your chances of falling.

Tip 95. Consider installing these devices in your house. Adaptive devices can help you to function and live easier in your house. Here are some suggestions.
    If you have trouble walking, you should put grab bars:

- On the walls near stairs and entranceways.

- On long hallway walls.
- In the bathroom near the tub and toilet.

If you have trouble getting out of bed, you should:

- Put bed rails on the bed.
- Move the bed against the wall and put a grab bar on that wall. Pull on the grab to rollover or get out of bed.
- Attach an overhead grab bar to a hospital bed. They are not the most attractive items, but they make it easier to move or rollover in bed.

If you have trouble eating, you should:

- Try using a child's snorkel style cup for drinking liquids.
- Use plates with divided sections. It easier to scoop food using the dividers than a flat style plate.
- Use plates with suction holders. They hold the plate firmly on the table, which makes cutting food easier.
- Wrap a facecloth around fork or spoon handles to make them easier to grab and hold. Secure the facecloth with tape.

Try these miscellaneous adaptive devices:

- Use touch style lights instead of lamps with small turn on dials.
- Use "clap on" devices.
- Buy an "over the bed" style table to use in your living room.
- Buy reach bars. A reach bar looks like big tweezers and allows you to pick up items off the floor without bending.
- Buy pencil grips at the stationary store and put them on crochet hooks, toothbrushes, or other small handles. The grips make it easier to hold and use these items.
- Buy special door handle covers that fit over your existing doorknobs to make opening doors easier.
- Change twisting style door handles to lever style handles. Opening doors will be much easier!

Devices are available to help you put on your shoes, slip on nylons, button your buttons, or even squeeze the toothpaste tube. You can find adaptive devices in pharmacies, hardware stores, or local medical supply stores. *Do not stop looking until you find the device you need.*

Tip 96. Consider buying a medical alert system. A medical alert system allows you to activate help quickly by simply pushing a button. The button is commonly worn on a chain around your neck. It allows you to call for help if you fall and are unable to reach the telephone. These systems vary in cost. Before buying a system, you should:

- Read the contract carefully. Ask a family to read through the contract.

- Ask the salesman if the unit can be rented instead of being bought. It may be cheaper to rent the unit.

- Ask the salesman to explain the maintenance contract.

- Ask the salesman how often they will test the system. It is important to have the system tested periodically to be sure it is properly working.

- Ask the salesman about their back up plans for power outages.

Internet Resources

- Go to the Visiting Nurse Association (www.vnaa.org) web site for information on finding and selecting a visiting nurse association. The site also has information on the types of services available and reimbursement details.

- Go to the American Physical Therapist Association (www.apta.org) web site and explore the information under "for consumers." It will give you information about physical therapy and how it can help you.

- Go to the America Occupational Therapist Association (www.aota.org) web site for some great tips and suggestions for living with specific disorders, such as, arthritis.

- Go to the American Speech and Hearing Association (www.asha.org) web site for help with hearing or speech problems. You can search their database for a pathologist near you.

- Value Care by Enrichments offers a large variety of devices. Call for a catalog (1-800-323-5547) or go to their web site at www.

<u>sammonspreston.com</u> for more information. They will assist you in billing Medicare for certain devices.

- Go to a search engine and type in these words: cane, walker, assistive devices, adaptive devices, physical or occupational therapy.

8

Infection Control:
"Should I get the flu vaccine?"
"How can I avoid getting a cold?"

Just the Facts

A bug is a microorganism that enters your body and causes an illness. Microorganisms can be bacterial or viral. Bacterial bugs cause diseases, such as, pneumonia, sinusitis, tonsillitis, and urinary tract infections. Antibiotics kill bacteria. Viral bugs cause diseases like the common cold. Antibiotics do *not* kill viruses.

🔑 Contrary to popular belief, hospitals are not pristine sterile facilities. They harbor and grow some of the most dangerous microorganisms. Nosocomial means an infection that was acquired within a hospital. Hospitals are required to monitor and track all nosocomial infections. Protect yourself from getting nosocomial infections by being proactive. If you become hospitalized, do *not* allow anyone (doctor, nurse, therapist) to perform any procedure on you unless they have *just* washed their hands and donned a *new* pair of gloves. Simply say, "Before changing my dressing, please wash your hands." Do not be intimidated to request a room change if your roommate is coughing or has diarrhea. These two symptoms can easily spread microorganisms. Protect yourself! You are in charge of your health care.

The Dreaded Flu

Influenza, also known as the flu, is a very contagious disease caused by a virus. It has been present for decades. In 1918, the Spanish Flu killed more than twenty million people. In 1957 and 1968, the Asian and Hong Kong flu's killed hundreds of thousands of people. About thirty six thousand people die each year from the flu and about one hundred thousand people are admitted into hospitals. These statistics are nothing to sneeze at! Unfortunately only ten to twenty percent of the population will get the flu vaccine each year.

The flu causes respiratory system problems. This means problems with the nose, throat, and lungs. It is very different than the common cold. Flu symptoms include:

- Fever.

- Fatigue.

- Headache.

- Dry cough.

- Sore throat.

- Nasal congestion.

- Body aches.

The most common complications are pneumonia, sinusitis, bronchitis, and related ear infections. It usually takes one to two weeks to recover from the flu.

The flu season is from November to March with January and February being the peak months. Coughing, speaking, and sneezing spreads it from person to person. When the virus enters your nose or mouth it begins to multiply. You will feel sick within one to four days.

If you get the flu, you should: get plenty of rest, drink a lot of fluids, avoid smoking, and take over the counter medications to help alleviate the symptoms. Your doctor may prescribe one of these antiviral medications:

- Tamiflu is an antiviral medication that helps to treat the flu and should be started within forty-eight hours of the onset of the flu symptoms. It is not a replacement for the annual flu shot. It may be taken with or without meals. If you develop a stomach upset, take the medication with food.

- Flumadine is used to treat influenza A and should be started within twenty-four to forty-eight hours after the onset of symptoms. Aspirin and acetaminophen interact with this medication and should *not* be taken concurrently. Take it several hours before bedtime to help prevent insomnia. Dizziness, headache, and fatigue are potential side effects so avoid driving or other hazardous activities.

- Relenza is an inhaled flu medication. Follow the instructions on the package for the proper method of loading the Diskhaler. It should be used cautiously with anyone who has respiratory diseases, such as, asthma or emphysema. If you normally use a bronchodilator inhaler, use that inhaler first and then the Relenza inhaler.

- Symmetrel is another flu medication, but it should be used cautiously in older people if heart, liver, or kidney disease is present. Take this medication a few hours before bedtime to prevent insomnia. If you develop dizziness, depression, anxiety, or any changes in your mental focus, call your doctor. Do not consume alcohol while taking this medication.

- Zinc, Echinacea, and vitamin C may help to reduce the severity or length of the flu.

All cough medicines do not act the same way. Use an expectorant cough medicine if you have a productive cough, lots of phlegm, or mucus in the lungs. An expectorant will get the congestion out of the lungs. Use a suppressant cough medicine to stop coughing. This medication should be used at night time or when there is no congestion. Follow the directions on the bottle. Never take more than the prescribed amount. If your coughing does not improve or lessen within a few days, seek medical attention. A prolonged chest cold can lead to pneumonia. *Pneumonia is a leading cause of death in older people.* If you have diabetes, look for cough syrups that are sugar, dextrose, and glycerin free. If you are taking any other medications that can cause drowsiness, you should avoid cough syrups containing alcohol.

Tip Exploration

Tip 97. Hand washing is the best way to control the spread of infections. Even with all the expensive antibiotics and treatments available, the simple step of hand washing is the most important! How long should hand washing last? It takes fifteen seconds to *properly* wash your hands. Most people wash their hands in less than ten seconds! Start by getting your hands soapy and then apply friction by rubbing your hands together. Be sure to wash between your fingers and around the cuticles. Dry your hands on a towel and then use the towel to turn off the faucet. If you touch the dirty faucet with your clean hands, you have defeated the purpose of hand washing. The faucet is dirty.

You are probably thinking, "This is so basic that it can not be important." You are very wrong. Did you know that hospital personnel are taught how to wash their hands? Hospitals hire special nurses to monitor the hospital's infection rate and the staff's hand washing skills. *Numerous studies have proven that hand washing is the single most effective way to prevent disease transmission.*

Wash your hands for fifteen seconds! _____

Place a √ mark when done.

Tip 98. Use caution with antibacterial soap. The advertisements sound great, but the using these soaps repetitively can cause microorganisms to be become stronger and more immune to antibiotics. If you choose to use them, alternate the brands and use them at only one sink. Use regular soap at the other sink.

Tip 99. Get your flu shot every year. The Centers for Disease Control and Prevention monitors the types of viruses most likely to infect people each year. They select some strains and begin to make the vaccine by putting the strains into chicken eggs where they will grow and multiply. After growing, the virus is killed and the vaccine is made from this dead material.

If you are allergic to egg products, you should *not* get the flu vaccine because it is grown inside eggs. It may be possible to receive the flu vaccine by going to an allergist. He will administer the vaccine in smaller doses over a longer period of time.

Get the flu vaccine as early possible because it takes about three weeks for your body to grow antibodies. Try to get the vaccine in October or November. Most senior centers run free flu clinics. While we are on the subject, I can hear someone saying, "The flu vaccine makes me sick." *The vaccine is not a live virus.* You can not get a cold or flu from the vaccine. The most common side effects from the vaccine include:

- Sore arm at the injection site.
- Low-grade fever.
- Tired and worn out feeling.
- Generalized muscle aches.

Tip 100. Tell your family members to get the flu vaccine. If your family members are in close contact with you, especially during the flu season, they should get the vaccine.

The Centers for Disease Control and Prevention recommends these people get the flu vaccine:

- Anyone over sixty-five years old.

- Residents of a nursing home or anyone who regularly visits a nursing home.

- Adults or child with heart, lung, or other chronic problems.

- Anyone with an immune compromised system.

- Women who will be in their second or third trimester of pregnancy.

- Health care workers.

- Anyone who lives with someone with an above condition.

The nasal flu vaccine, which is administered by nose drops, can only be given to people between the ages of five and fifty because the vaccine is administered live.

Tip 101. Get the pneumonia vaccine. The pneumonia vaccine is different than the flu vaccine. It is generally given free and at flu clinics. In most cases, you will only need to get it once in your lifetime. Pneumonia is a leading cause of death among older Americans. Prevention is the number one goal.

Tip 102. Keep all immunizations up to date. As we get older, we forget about getting regular immunizations. Tetanus is fairly rare disease, however the majority of people who die from it are over sixty years old! Get a tetanus immunization every ten years.

Hepatitis B immunizations are encouraged for certain people. Hepatitis B is a serious disease that results in liver inflammation and can lead to death. You should get this vaccine if you:

- Had a blood transfusion between 1978–1985.

- Worked as a healthcare worker.

- Participated in homosexual relationships.

- Worked as a prostitute.

- Used illegal drugs.

Get a PPD test done to check for exposure to tuberculosis. Tuberculosis is a serious lung disease that is on the rise in the United States. A PPD test is recommended for anyone:

- Working in a health care setting.

- Working or visiting prisons on a regular basis.

- Working or visiting nursing homes on a regular basis.

- Traveling to or having visitors from foreign countries where tuberculosis is common.

Tip 103. Look for signs of an infection. All wounds heal differently. The speed at which your wound heals depends on the type of injury, seriousness, and your overall health. Wounds heal best when they are clean and kept dry. Wash all wounds with soap and water. Put a clean bandage or dressing on them. Watch for signs of infection including:

- Redness or a red streak coming from the wound.

- Warmth at the wound site.

- Low grade fever.

- Increased in pain at the wound site.

- Drainage from the wound.

- Odor from the wound.

If you notice any signs of an infection, call your doctor or go to the emergency room.

Internet Resources

- Go the Center for Disease Control and Prevention (www.cdc.gov) web site for information about the flu and the flu vaccine. The site also has information about other communicable diseases and prevention tips.

- The National Coalition for Adult Immunizations (www.nfid.org/ncai) web site for more information about adult immunizations.

- Go to a search engine and type these words: flu, influenza, infection, immunizations, tuberculosis, hepatitis, and pneumonia.

9

Legal Concerns:
"What is a living will?"
"How do I create one?"

Just the Facts

The hospital is required by law to give you various pieces of paper upon admission. It is important to read these papers thoroughly. Hospitals will give you information about "your bill of rights" and "advance directives." Here is an explanation of these two items.

Bill of Rights

The American Hospital Association created a patient's Bill of Rights to ensure all patients are treated fairly and equally. You need to know your rights! Here is a summary of them:

- You have the right to considerate and respectful care.
- You have the right to know your diagnosis, treatment, and prognosis.
- You have the right to know the identity of the staff taking care of you.
- You have the right to make decisions about your care. You can refuse care to the extent that is allowed by your states laws.
- You have the right to create an advance directive.
- You have the right to privacy. You have the right to expect that your medical records and personal information will be kept confidential.
- You have the right to review your medical record.

- You have the right to accept or decline participation in any research program.

- You have the right to be transferred to another facility when is determined to be medically and legally permissible.

- You have the right to be informed about various policies and procedures that affect your care. You have the right to information about filing grievances and conflict resolution.

- You have the right to be informed about hospital charges and payment options.

If you feel your rights have been violated, call the hospital and speak to administrative personnel. Go to the American Hospital Association (www.aha.org) web site for more information about your health care rights and filing grievances.

Advance Directive

The hospital admitting staff must ask you if you have an advance directive. If you have one, you will be asked to bring a copy of it to the hospital. If you do not have an advance directive, you will be given papers explaining them and a template to complete one if you choose.

An advance directive is a legal document that explains your wishes regarding end of life care issues. Advance directives consist of two parts: the living will and the health care surrogate.

Living Will

A living will focuses on meeting your wishes while you are alive. It allows you to specify how much medical care you want to take place on your behalf, in case you are *unable* to verbalize these wishes. A living will should address your feelings on whether or not you would want these four things done to you:

1. If your heart stopped, would you want cardiopulmonary resuscitation (CPR) started?

2. If you were unable to breathe on your own, would you want to be put on a respirator (breathing machine)?

3. If you were unable to eat food on your own, would you want to be fed through a stomach tube?

4. If your kidneys stopped working, would you want to be put on a dialysis machine?

You can say yes to some actions and no to other ones. It is your decision. It is perfectly fine to say, "I want everything done," or "I want nothing done." *Never be coerced into signing a document in which you do not feel comfortable.* I encourage you to speak to your doctor about these choices. They can explain the pros and cons of each intervention based on your medical problems.

If you create an advance directive, you will still receive pain medications and other appropriate interventions. Creating an advance directive does *not* mean that you will be left to die or given medications to die. It is not a suicide wish or statement.

Health Care Surrogate

The second part of an advance directive is assigning someone to be your health care agent or surrogate. *This person will communicate your wishes to the hospital staff and doctors if you are unable to do so.* Think of this person as your voice. Talk with your surrogate and explain your wishes. After your talk, ask yourself: "Are they comfortable with my wishes?" "Do they understand my wishes?" "Will they follow my wishes?"

Your surrogate does *not* have to believe in the same things that you do, but they should understand your wishes and feel comfortable following them. Sons or daughters are generally chosen to be surrogates. Clergy members, neighbors, or close friends may also be chosen. Your doctor can not be listed as your health care surrogate.

The Form

Complete the advance directive form after you have finalized your thoughts. Give a copy of the form to your doctor, health care surrogate, and appropriate family members.

Attorneys are usually not needed to complete this form, but if you have an attorney supply them with a copy of your directive. Each state has various laws concerning advance directives. Ask the hospital's admission staff or your doctor about your states specific laws.

There is no expiration date on advance directives. If you decide to change your wishes, simply tear up the form and create a new one. Make sure the date is clearly written on the new form and notify both your doctor and health care surrogate.

$\mathcal{P}$ Cardiopulmonary Resuscitation (CPR) is an emergency procedure that can save your life. CPR is started when you have a cardiac arrest. A cardiac arrest means that your heart and breathing have stopped. A trained person will blow oxygen into your mouth by sealing their lips onto yours. Various mouth devices are used inside hospitals. Someone will also push down on your breastbone to circulate your blood. CPR does not always restart your heart. Medications and defibrillation may also be needed.

Traditional Will

A traditional will is a legal document that describes who will get your property or other assets and who will manage your estate after you die. A probate hearing will be scheduled to determine how your estate is divided. Your will is read during the probate hearing. If you do not have a will, the court will assign an administrator to determine the value of your estate and recommend how it should be divided.

It is best to seek legal advice to create a traditional will. There are also many Internet sites available to assist you in creating a will. Go to www.legalzoom.com for a comprehensive legal web site and get more information about completing a will online.

Tip Exploration

Tip 104. Talk to your family about your advance directive. It is very difficult to initiate this conversation, but chances are your sons or daughters have wondered about your wishes. Often they feel uncomfortable approaching the subject with you. From a daughter's perspective and from years of nursing experiences, I can tell you that it is better to know someone's wishes ahead of time than to have to make a quick decision inside a hospital setting.

Tell your family that you want to discuss your will and advance directive. Plan a convenient date and time for the meeting. Preplanning a date allows your family time to process their thoughts and feelings. Most hospitals and doctor offices have pamphlets available that explain these issues in detail. Have the pamphlets available at the meeting. Young children should not be present because it may confuse and scare them.

Tell your family how you feel about having CPR performed or being put on a breathing machine. Reassure them that you have given a lot of thought to your decision. Allow family members time to express their thoughts and concerns.

Family meeting date set. _____

Place a √ mark when done.

Tip 105. Discuss your feelings and thoughts about funeral or burial plans. This is also a very difficult discussion to start, but it is very important. Being open and honest about your wishes will help your family members through a difficult time. Tell them where cemetery deeds are stored. Discuss your feelings on cremation and church services. If you have prepaid your funeral expenses, make sure your family knows this information. Prepaying funeral expenses has certain tax advantages. Ask an accountant to discuss the advantages.

Tip 106. Create a traditional will and discuss it with your family. It is important to ask your sons or daughters for input regarding your estate. Maybe your daughter adores a particular piece of jewelry or your son wants a particular picture. An open and honest discussion about these issues will prevent sibling rivalry or hard feelings later.

Will created and discussed with family. _____

Place a √ mark when done.

Tip 107. Complete an anatomical gift card. An anatomical gift card expresses your wishes to give part or all of your body for research, transplantation, medical or dental education, or to the advancement of science. You can request that only a particular body part be given or you can donate your entire body. Older people with medical problems can still donate body parts, such as, eyes, skin, and bones. You can select who can receive this gift. For example, it may a hospital, medical school or organ procurement organization. This gift can be written into your living will or can be created separately. Tell your doctor and health care surrogate about these wishes. You can change your gift card wishes at any time. This is truly the gift that keeps on giving!

Anatomical gift card created. _____

Place a √ mark when done.

Internet Resources

- Go to the Legal Zoom (www.Legalzoom.com) web site for information about various legal issues. You can submit personal questions that will be answered in a timely manner.

- Go to the Legal Forms (<u>www.Findlegalforms.com</u>) web site for a selection of various legal documents and forms that can be printed and completed.

- Go to the Organ Donor (<u>www.Organdonor.org</u>) web site for information on organ donation. You can get a donor card from the site.

- Go to the Medem (<u>www.medem.com</u>) web site for information and guidance about "end of life care" issues. Medem is a site full of other health care issues and information.

- Go to a search engine and type these words: legal, legal forms, wills, advance directives, end of life care, and organ donation.

10

Frequently Asked Questions

Your Questions

Throughout my nursing career, I have been asked many questions. Here are some frequently asked questions and responses.

"I do not think I am getting the best medical care. Should I see a specialist? If I want a second opinion, will my primary doctor be upset? If you do not feel you are getting the best care, or if you want a second opinion, then by all means get it! A good doctor will *never* be upset if you choose to get another opinion. Actually most doctors would encourage you to get a second opinion. A specialist would be the most logical next choice. Depending on your insurance, a referral may be needed from your primary doctor. Depending on the specialty and nature of the medical problem, it may take a few weeks to get an appointment with a specialist.

What is the difference between a nursing home and an assisted living facility? A new wave of medical care facilities has erupted called assisted living facilities. There is a big difference between a nursing home and an assisted living facility. A nursing home (skilled nursing facility, convalescent home) is staffed twenty-four hours per day with nurses. Other staff will include various therapists, dietary personnel, and nursing assistants. A doctor will be in charge of the facility. All nursing homes are visited and licensed by the individual state's health department. Call the health department to review their inspection records for any outstanding violations.

An assisted living facility is similar to living in an apartment complex except that some medical care is offered. The facilities vary, but most will have a nursing department that can assist you with dressing changes, medications, and certain therapies. Nurses are usually only present during daytime hours. Most facilities will provide two or three prepared meals per day that are eaten in a main dining room. Most apartments will be one-bedroom units with a small efficiency style kitchen. Social activities will be planned throughout the day. An assisted living facility may be an ideal option for you. You will not have the expense and up keep of a private house and yard. Before signing a contract to move in, you should:

- Attend a few social functions.
- Eat in the dinning room. Look at copies of their menus.
- Ask about their transportation services.
- Ask about their security systems.
- Ask about their policies regarding pets and visitors.
- Read *all* of their policies.

Make sure you are comfortable with your decision. Do not feel pressured or pushed into making a quick decision. Give yourself time to think about it. This is a big decision!

"Should I buy long term care insurance?" The average monthly cost for a nursing home is about four thousand eight hundred dollars per month. This number varies based on where you live. Insurance plans are available to help you cover the expense of a nursing home beyond the amount that Medicare or your other health insurance covers. Before signing for an expensive policy, ask yourself a few questions:

- "If I am unable to live alone, can I live with my family?"
- "What types of heath care problems do I have?"
- "What is my long term prognosis?" (Speak to your doctor).
- "Can I afford to pay the premiums?" *Your premiums should not exceed seven percent of your annual income.*
- "Should I save the money from the premiums and use it for home care help?"

Assume your monthly income is three thousand eight hundred dollars. Can you afford to pay the difference of one thousand dollars per month (assuming that the nursing home bill is four thousand eight hundred dollars)? Long term care insurance premiums can cost a few hundred dollars per month to over a thousand. You can reduce the premium by purchasing insurance that only pays the difference between your monthly income and the monthly cost of a nursing home.

The length of the policy is another way to lower your premiums. Some policies will provide you with long term care insurance for three or five year periods instead of a lifetime. Lifetime policies are the most expensive. Look at your overall health and age and then make a smart consumer decision. For example, if you are seventy-five years old and have numerous health care problems, a five or ten year policy may make more sense than a lifetime policy.

Carefully read the policy before signing. Ask your son or daughter to review it Follow your gut instinct and beware of scam artists. Never buy a policy from a stranger at your door. Start by asking your home or car insurance agent for a policy and quote.

"I am scared that someday I will wake up and find her dead. What should I do if that happens?" This is a common fear that many spouses or family members share when they live with someone with multiple medical problems. You will need to call your local emergency medical services number. The dispatcher will ask you some basic information. Depending on your state's laws an ambulance service and or a police officer will be sent to the house. They will ask you information about her health and then call her doctor. Depending on the circumstances, your loved one would then be sent to a funeral home. If you have a "Do Not Resuscitate" medical order completed, your health care provider will give additional instructions to you.

Do not remove any medical devices that are attached to the deceased until emergency personnel arrive. If you suspect that your family member has committed suicide, do not touch anything in the house or move the body. Leave everything as is and call your local emergency medical services number.

"Is pain a normal experience for older people?" No! Pain is a symptom of a problem. New therapies have emerged to control pain even in severe cases. Most large cities have pain clinics offering various treatment options. Get the relief you need and deserve!

"I have heard about the vial of life. What is it?" The vial of life is a "test tube" like container that holds important health information including: your doctor's name, medication list, allergies, medical and surgical history, and next of kin information. The vial is stored in the refrigerator on the door shelf. The kit comes with two stickers. Place one sticker on your front door and the other one on the refrigerator door. Ambulance personnel are trained to look for the sticker and vial. It can provide them with key information in the event that you are unable to provide the information. Call your local visiting nurse association or emergency service department to obtain a vial. If they do not have them, go online and use a search engine. Type the phrase "vial of life." They are generally free to senior citizens!

"How do we get a hospital bed into the house?" Great question! First and foremost have the doctor order the bed for medical reasons. Your health insurance will then pay for it. Be sure to order an electric style bed. If possible, opt for a bed with both adjustable legs and head sections. These beds allow for easier body positioning. Ask the vendor if they can supply two or three fitted sheets. Your regular fitted sheets may be too small to tightly fit over the mattress. Order an egg crate mattress pad at the same time. The egg crate mattress pad is a foam pad that goes between the mattress and the sheet. It helps to provide protection to the skin.

Before the bed arrives, give some thought to where you want it set up. It should be close to the bathroom and on the main floor of the house. Sometimes families like to place the bed in the living room so that the person is not "left out". Use your best judgement. If there are small children or frequent visitors, put the bed in a side room. This allows for privacy and for periods of rest.

"My bed is an electric hospital bed. What happens when the power goes out?" Power outages can occur anywhere, anytime, and to any household. Start by calling your electric supply company and ask for their emergency plan support personnel. Explain your situation. Ask them what the emergency plan is for your area. Most companies have a priority list of homes that need to have power restored quickly due to medical conditions. Most power companies will require a form to be completed and signed by the doctor.

Even if your name is on the list, there is no guarantee power will be restored quickly. You need a back up plan. Know the locations of emergency shelters, hours of operation, and contact phone numbers. If you live where frequent evacuations occur, hurricanes or floods, have a plan in place. Call your local American Red Cross chapter or visit their web site (www.redcross.org) for preparation guidelines. *You can not prevent the power outages, but you can be prepared for them!*

"I am on oxygen and afraid to go anywhere. Can I leave my house?" Absolutely, you can leave the house! It is important to remain as active as possible. Call for a "Breathin' Easy" travel guide. The telephone number is 888-699-4360 or you can visit their web site at www.breathineasy.com. This guide will give you important safety tips about traveling with an oxygen tank. If you are planning to travel by airplane, you need to do some preplanning. Start by calling your airline. *You will not be allowed to use your oxygen tank during the flight.* Most airlines will supply an oxygen tank for you during the flight for an additional cost. However, some airlines have limits on the liters per minute that can be used. The cost of oxygen ranges from fifty to one hundred and fifty dollars per flight. You will need a doctor's prescription. The prescription must include this information:

- Name, address, and telephone number of the doctor.
- The number of flow liters per minute at altitude of eight thousand feet.
- Duration that the oxygen will be needed.
- Method for using the oxygen (cannula or mask).

In addition, some airlines require specific forms and liability releases to be signed. Most airlines will allow you to ship *empty* tanks and respiratory equipment as baggage. You must make arrangements for your tanks to be filled once you get to your destination. Call your airline at least one month ahead of time to finalize arrangements. Amtrak does allow oxygen tanks to be used on the train. Call Amtrak directly for more information and charges.

"How do I get a handicapped sticker for my car?" Start by calling your local department of motor vehicles. In most states, a doctors signature will be required stating that you have limited mobility due to a medical condition. Some states require that these stickers be renewed every year while other states have longer expiration times.

"I have a glass thermometer at home. Can I still use it?" The old style glass thermometers contain mercury. It is best *not* to use them; instead purchase a digital oral thermometer. They are very inexpensive and can be bought in most pharmacies.

You may remember playing with mercury balls during your childhood, but they actually pose an environmental threat and a health risk. Mercury filled thermometers that break or are thrown away can leak mercury into the environment during the incineration process. The amount of mercury may seem insignificant, but multiply your small amount by your neighbors and their neighbors, and so on.

If your thermometer breaks at home and you see mercury, follow these clean up steps:

- Do not use household cleaning products with ammonia or chloride to clean the spill. They will interact and create toxic fumes.
- Do not use your vacuum cleaner. Vacuums will put the mercury vapor into the air and increase the potential dangers.
- Do not use a broom because it can break the mercury into smaller pieces and spread them out more.

- Use eyedroppers to pick up the pieces or scoop them with a heavy piece of paper. Place the droppers, papers, thermometer parts, and the mercury into a plastic bag and seal it tight. Double and triple bag it. Call your local waste department for disposal instructions.

- If the weather permits, leave your windows open for at least one day.

- Check out the Environmental Protection Agency (www.epa.gov) web site for more information.

Family Member Questions

Family members and other caregivers have asked me many questions. Here are some of your frequently asked questions and responses.

"Can I buy the hospital style patient gowns for my mom?" Yes. Hospital style gowns have many benefits for people with limited mobility. They are easily laundered, durable, and allow for basic hygiene tasks to be easily performed. They come in numerous fabrics and patterns that disguise them from the institutional look. You can order them through pharmacies or on the Internet.

"How can I get any rest when I am caring for my mom twenty-fours a day?" Being the primary caregiver is very difficult. Start with your local visiting nurse organization. Most of these agencies have home health aides or homemakers that can help relieve some of the burden. Local temporary nursing agencies may also be helpful. Be careful when hiring someone directly from the newspaper. Check all references and be sure that they are bonded.

"My mother cannot be left alone for more than a few hours. How can we go away on a vacation without her?" Most assisted living facilities or hospice units will have respite care capabilities. Respite care allows the "sick" person to be cared for by professional medical personnel for a limited time. Depending on the medical condition, some insurance companies will pay for part or all of the respite care. Make arrangements early. Her doctor can give you additional tips and recommendations.

It is important for you to know that hospice is not just for cancer patients. Hospice services can help any person regardless of age or diagnosis if their condition is determined to be terminal or not treatable. Medicare has special benefits available to patients enrolled in hospice care. These benefits cover respite care.

Go to the National Family Caregiver's Association (www.nfcacares.org) web site for some additional ideas and support systems for you. Also, check out the Visiting Nurse Association (www.vnaa.org) web site for caregiver support systems.

"My dad wanted me to take him to the cemetery to place flowers at mom's grave site. Is that normal? Should I take him?" Visiting a spouse's gravesite is normal. It can help with the grieving process. Anniversary dates and holidays are often the most difficult and visiting the cemetery may be reassuring. *The loss of a spouse is a monumental event in your dad's life.* Sadness is a normal reaction. There is no time frame for grieving or being sad.

However, depression is very different. Depression is a medical condition that needs professional help. The signs of depression include:

- A change in sleeping patterns; either sleeping too little or too much.

- A change in appetite; either an increased or decreased appetite.

- Loss of interest or pleasure in activities once enjoyed.

- Inabilities to concentrate, remember basic information, or make decisions.

- Unexplained fatigue or loss of energy.

- Expressions of guilt, hopelessness, or worthlessness.

- A sudden increase in complaints including: headaches, chronic pains, or body aches without a definitive cause.

If you see these signs or remain concerned about your dad's mental health, speak to his doctor. Your dad is not alone. According to the National Institute of Health, about one in every five people will suffer depression at sometime during their life. In most cases, it can be handled with medications. It is important not to ignore the symptoms. Untreated depression can lead to malnutrition, failure to thrive syndrome, and even suicide.

"I do not think that she is a safe driver. What can I do about her driving a car?" This is perhaps one of the toughest questions that face older Americans. A driver's license symbolizes freedom and youth. Taking away someone's ability to drive is often heart wrenching for everyone involved. Here are a few suggestions:

- Encourage your mother to take a driver's update course. The AARP offers them in most states.

- Discuss your concerns with your mother in a friendly, supportive manner. Listen to her concerns and accept her fears. Do not be judgmental. Avoid phrases like, "You are too old to drive," instead say, "How can I help you with your errands?"

- Offer solutions to limit her driving. For example, take her shopping, make her doctor and hair appointments at times when you could drive.

- Look in the newspaper for advertisements for transportation. Place an advertisement yourself under "help wanted."

- Obtain bus schedules from senior or community centers.

- Agree on driving limits. For example, only drive during daytime hours, set a mileage limit, agree to no highway driving.

- If these tips do not work and you mother is a driving danger, you need to contact your states motor vehicle department. It is important to protect her and the public's safety.

"The nurse at the hospital told my dad that he could not drive because he had a seizure. Is that true?" Yes. Most states have laws that mandate how long someone must be "seizure free" to resume driving. Failure to comply with these laws can result in fines and loss of the driver's license. Some insurance companies have additional rules that will need to be followed.

Internet Resources

There are many Internet resources available to help you. Start with these sites:

- Go to the Family Care Giver Alliance (www.caregiver.org) web site for information about various resources and support programs.

- Go to the Elder Care www.eldercare.com web site for a lot of helpful information. You will find legal and financial information, advice on hiring home care helpers, and other resource information.

- Go to the National Association for Homecare (www.nahc.org) web site for advice and guidance on hiring and finding homecare assistance.

- Go to a search engine and type these words: caregiver, eldercare, support services and, homecare.

Take care of yourself. Being a caregiver is hard work. It often is a juggling act between your personal life, work, kids, and a sick family member. Take care of yourself first. Eat right, exercise, and get plenty of sleep. You will *not* be an effective caregiver when you are exhausted and worn out. Trust me, I have been there. Take a few minutes every day to recharge your battery. Learn to say no. For example, "No, I can not make cupcakes for the scout meeting." *If you try to be a superhero to every one all the time, you will not be a hero to anyone.* Treat yourself to a bubble bath, dinner out, a new book, or something that help you to relax and rejuvenate. There is a light at the end of the tunnel.

Running errands for your parents can be exhausting, frustrating, and even aggravating at times. Try to cherish those moments with your mom or dad. If you are taking them grocery shopping, stop and have a cup of coffee together. You will feel better in the long run, again, just trust me. Life is to short.

Someday you may need to place a parent into a nursing home. It is normal to have feelings of guilt and sadness. However, it is also normal to feel a sense of relief and freedom. That sense of relief often triggers guilt feelings. Do not hide your emotions. Let the tears flow. Do not try to stop them. The tears are part of the healing process. As the song words from the musical Annie say, "The sun will come out tomorrow."

APPENDIX A

Preventive Medicine Checklist

Place a check mark next to the screening tests that you have completed. Schedule the unmarked tests with your doctor.

Screening tests for everyone:

- ❑ See the dentist twice a year. Ask the dentist to look for signs of oral cancer.

- ❑ Get an eye exam. Ask the doctor to do a glaucoma screening, starting at age sixty-five. If you have diabetes, are of African American decent, or if your parents had glaucoma, testing should be started at age forty.

- ❑ Professional hearing test. This should be done annually starting at age sixty-five.

- ❑ Blood pressure. At minimum, this should be done annually starting at age forty-five.

- ❑ Bone density. This should be done annually starting at age sixty-five.

- ❑ Colon cancer screening. This consists of a colonoscopy and should be done annually starting at age fifty.

- ❑ Complete skin evaluation. Your doctor should closely examine your scalp, back, arms, legs, and chest for possible signs of skin cancer.

- ❑ Blood test for cholesterol. This should be done every five years starting at age thirty-five.

Specific screening test for men:

❑   Prostate screening. This should be done annually starting at age fifty. This may consist of blood work, prostate specific antigen (PSA), or a digital rectal examination.

Specific screening tests for women:

❑   Self breast examinations. This should be done monthly. Do not stop because your menses have stopped. Have an annual breast examination by your doctor.

❑   Mammogram. This should be done annually starting at age forty or earlier based on family history.

❑   Pap test. This should be done every three years.

APPENDIX B

Doctor's Appointment Checklist

Make copies of this sheet to bring to your doctor's appointments. Place a check mark next to the items you want to discuss with the doctor.

Bring these items with you:

- ❏ Medication chart. Ask: Can I stop taking any of these medications? Am I taking the right dosage? What is this pill for? What are its side effects? Does this pill interact with any foods?

- ❏ Bring any over the counter medications. Ask: Are these safe to take? Will these interact with my prescription medications? How often can I take them?

- ❏ Bring any herbal supplements with you. Ask: Are these safe to take? Do they work? Do they interact with my prescription medications? How often can I take them?

- ❏ If you are a diabetic, bring your glucometer or a record of your blood sugar tests.

- ❏ Other:

Other questions to ask your doctor:

- ❏ What type of diet should I be on?

- ❏ Do you want me to have any blood tests done? Cholesterol, blood sugar, general panel (hemoglobin, hematocrit, electrolytes), therapeutic drug levels.

- ❏ What was my blood pressure? _____Is this a safe range for me?

- ❏ Are there any alternative treatments that I should try?

❑   When is my next appointment?

❑   Other:

Tell your doctor:

❑   If you have fallen since your last visit.

❑   About any dizziness or headaches that you have experienced since your last visit.

❑   If you have had any chest pain, chest tightness, or trouble breathing.

❑   If you have noticed any vision changes.

❑   If you have noticed any hearing changes.

❑   If you have noticed any bowel changes.

❑   If you are having any urinary incontinence problems.

❑   If you have sores or wounds that are not healing.

❑   About any pain that you are experiencing.

❑   Other:

APPENDIX C

Questions to Ask Your Surgeon

Ask the surgeon these questions before agreeing to surgery. Bring a family member with you. Never feel pressured or be coerced into having surgery. A good surgeon will take the time needed to answer your questions. There are situations that require immediate surgical intervention and timing may not allow for all of these questions to be answered.

- ❑ What is the name of the operation? Make sure that he gives you the technical name and then defines it in terms that you understand. For example, if the surgeon says, "you need a cholecystectomy," the surgeon should explain to you that this is the removal of the gallbladder.

- ❑ Why do I need to have this surgery?

- ❑ Are there any alternatives to this surgery? For examples, gallstones can sometimes be chemically dissolved.

- ❑ Can this surgery be done using laparoscopic techniques? This involves a small instrument that is inserted through a tiny incision into your body.

- ❑ What are the benefits to having this surgery? What are the risks? What are the odds of these risks? Every surgery, no matter how minor, comes with some risks.

- ❑ How big will the incision be? Where will it be? Will there be more than one incision?

- ❑ Who will be assisting you? Most surgeries require the surgeon to have an assistant. You should know who it is and their qualifications.

- ❑ What has been your experience doing this surgery? How many of these surgeries do you do every year?

❑   Will this surgery have an effect on my other medical problems?

❑   Should I continue to my medications? Tell the surgeon about any herbal supplements that you are taking.

❑   What type of anesthesia will I need? Some types completely put you to sleep and others have only a local reaction.

❑   Who will handle the anesthesia? Anesthesiologists are doctors; anesthetists are nurses.

❑   What is the anticipated recuperation time frame?

❑   Will my insurance pay for part or all of this surgery? Will anesthesia be covered by my insurance?

❑   Have you ever been suspended or lost your medical license? Most states have a web site that lists disciplinary actions taken against doctors. Check it out!

If you are not satisfied with the surgeon's answers, get a second opinion. It is your right!

Appendix D

Discharge Instructions

Before being discharged from the hospital, get the answers to these questions. If possible, have a family member present. Nurses are responsible for reviewing your discharge instructions. Clarify any information that is different from what your doctor told you. *Do not leave the hospital until you understand your instructions.*

Questions to ask the nurse:
General:

☐ When should I see my doctor again? Has an appointment been scheduled?

☐ How much walking can I do? Can I climb stairs?

☐ Can I drive my car?

☐ Can I take a bath or shower?

☐ How much weight can I lift?

☐ Should I expect any pain? How can I relieve the pain?

☐ If I develop problems, should I call my surgeon or my primary care doctor?

Medications:

☐ What medications should I take?

☐ When should I start taking them?

☐ Why do I need to take this medication? How does it work?

☐ What is the dosage of these medications?

☐ Are there any side effects to these medications?

☐ Are there any foods that interact with these medications?

☐ Do you have the prescriptions or have they been called them into the pharmacy?

Bandages or dressings:

☐ Should I change them?

☐ How often should the dressings be changed?

☐ Are there sutures (stitches) under the dressing? How many?

☐ When will these sutures be removed?

☐ Are there any drains or tubes under the dressing?

☐ How do I care for these drains or tubes?

☐ How much drainage can I expect to have from these tubes?

☐ How do I empty the drain container?

Other:

- If you need help at home, ask for it. Ask for a nurse, physical therapist, or occupational therapist referral. Ask for home health aides or a homemaker service. Be assertive. You are going to be very weak and tired once you get home. Do not over do it. Go slow. Get the help you need so that you can rest and get stronger.

APPENDIX E

Summary of the 107 Tips

Tip 1. Get a good doctor.

Tip 2. Make an appointment to see the doctor, dentist, eye doctor, and hearing specialist.

Tip 3. Learn from your past.

Tip 4. Allow extra time to gather thoughts and plan your day.

Tip 5. Be open to change.

Tip 6. Do not say the word, "never!"

Tip 7. Get a medical alert tag.

Tip 8. Create an emergency card for your wallet.

Tip 9. Keep on moving.

Tip 10. Make cheat notes!

Tip 11. Drink plenty of fluids especially water.

Tip 12. Apply sunscreens and wear broad rim hats when working in the yard.

Tip 13. Change your position slowly.

Tip 14. Wear shoes with laces and solid soles.

Tip 15. Obtain walking devices (canes, walkers) to help you.

Tip 16. Ask your doctor about medications to improve your balance and walking.

Tip 17. Keep areas brightly lit, but avoid glare.

Tip 18. Keep your hot water heater at 110° F (43° C) degrees.

Tip 19. Install smoke detectors and carbon monoxide detectors.

Tip 20. Choose the best floor covering.

Tip 21. Avoid climbing stairs.

Tip 22. No climbing on step stools!

Tip 23. Never use the oven or stove to heat your house.

Tip 24. Change your kitchen sponges at least once a month.

Tip 25. Replace your old knives with sharp new ones.

Tip 26. Do not smoke in bed.

Tip 27. Clear the hallway to the bathroom before going to sleep.
Tip 28. Keep a telephone by the bedside.
Tip 29. Install grab bars in the shower stall and near the toilet.
Tip 30. Get a raised toilet seat.
Tip 31. Use a shower chair instead of standing while showering.
Tip 32. Get motion sensor lights.
Tip 33. Know your limits.
Tip 34. Keep walkways clear of obstacles including snow, ice, and leaves.
Tip 35. Ask questions about your medications.
Tip 36. Organize your medications.
Tip 37. Buy all your prescriptions at one place.
Tip 38. Do not skip or double up on your medications.
Tip 39. Always finish your prescription.
Tip 40. Alcohol intake interacts with some medications.
Tip 41. Supplements can be beneficial, but some are very dangerous.
Tip 42. Seek financial resources for buying medications.
Tip 43. Use caution when buying medications on the Internet or from another country.
Tip 44. Get your blood tests done.
Tip 45. Keep medications in the correct bottles.
Tip 46. Do not break or crush medication pills.
Tip 47. Clean out your medicine cabinet.
Tip 48. Read food labels.
Tip 49. Make your plate look like a rainbow.
Tip 50. Limit your intake of canned foods and processed meats.
Tip 51. Use herbs or spices to add flavor to your food.
Tip 52. Try supplemental drinks.
Tip 53. Eat small and frequent meals.
Tip 54. Get good dental care.
Tip 55. Drink your milk!
Tip 56. Stop eating two hours before bedtime.
Tip 57. Use antacids with caution.
Tip 58. Explore new food cultures.
Tip 59. Share casseroles with neighbors or friends.
Tip 60. Keep it safe!
Tip 61. Be a savvy food shopper.
Tip 62. Make eating fun.
Tip 63. Allow yourself a treat.

Tip 64. Conserve energy by using ramekins.

Tip 65. Try non-medication treatments for digestive ulcers.

Tip 66. Talk to your doctor about medication options for digestive ulcers.

Tip 67. Try Kegel exercises for urinary incontinence problems.

Tip 68. Try bladder training exercises.

Tip 69. Talk to your doctor about pelvic floor treatments.

Tip 70. Talk to your doctor about medication options for urinary incontinence.

Tip 71. Treat constipation with good eating habits.

Tip 72. Use laxatives with caution.

Tip 73. Do not strain when having a bowel movement.

Tip 74. Stop diarrhea as soon as possible.

Tip 75. Try these tips to control gas problems.

Tip 76. Set goals.

Tip 77. Plan your reward.

Tip 78. Get a partner.

Tip 79. Plan your mental exercises.

Tip 80. Plan your social activities.

Tip 81. Volunteer for an organization.

Tip 82. Plan your physical exercises.

Tip 83. Get a pedometer.

Tip 84. Have a good laugh!

Tip 85. Buy good exercise equipment.

Tip 86. Form a telephone call tree system with your friends.

Tip 87. Return to school.

Tip 88. Get a pet.

Tip 89. Turn on the music!

Tip 90. Stop every fifteen minutes and drink a glass of water while exercising.

Tip 91. Obtain a referral from your doctor for the above health care professionals.

Tip 92. Do your homework before hiring private duty help.

Tip 93. Canes provide stability when walking.

Tip 94. Walkers provide a broader sense of stability when walking.

Tip 95. Consider installing these devices in your house.

Tip 96. Consider buying a medical alert system.

Tip 97. Hand washing is the best way to control the spread of infections.

Tip 98. Use caution with antibacterial soap.

Tip 99. Get your flu shot every year.

Tip 100. Tell your family members to get the flu vaccine.

Tip 101. Get the pneumonia vaccine.

Tip 102. Keep all immunizations up to date.

Tip 103. Look for signs of an infection.

Tip 104. Talk to your family about your advance directive.

Tip 105. Discuss your feelings and thoughts about funeral or burial plans.

Tip 106. Create a traditional will and discuss it with your family.

Tip 107. Complete an anatomical gift card.

Bibliography

- American Heart Association. *Heart disease and stroke statistics-2003 update.* Dallas, American Heart Association; 2003.

- Bates, DW, Spell, N, Cullen DJ, et al. The costs of adverse drug events in hospitalized patients. *JAMA.* 1997 (4): 307-11.

- Beers, MH, Berkow, R. *The Merck Manual of Geriatrics.* 3rd ed. West Point, PA: Merck Research Laboratories; 2000.

- Birge. SJ. Osteoporosis and hip fracture. *Clinical Geriatric Medicine.* 1993; 9(1): 69-71.

- Chan, FK, Leung, WK. Peptic-ulcer disease. *Lancet.* 2002; 360:933-941.

- Chapin, R, Dobbs-Kepper, D. Aging in place in assisted living: philosophy versus policy. *Gerontologist* 2001; 41(1): 43-50.

- Department of Health and Human Services. Centers for Medicare and Medicaid Services. Nursing Home Data Compendium 2000.

- Dowd T, et al. Using cognitive strategies to enhance bladder control and comfort. *Holistic Nurse Practice* 2000; 14(2): 19-103

- Eastell, R. Treatment of postmenopausal osteoporosis. *New England Journal of Medcine.*1995: 767-73.

- Eisenberg, D. Unconventional medicine in the United States-prevalence, costs, and patterns of use. *New England Journal of Medicine.* January 1993:246-252.

- Eisenberg, D. Trends in alternative medicine use in the United States. *JAMA.* 1998; 280:1569-1575.

- *Facts and Trends: the assisted living sourcebook.* Washington, DC: National Center for Assisted Living; 2001.

- Fultz, NH, Herzog, AR. Self reported social and emotional impact of urinary incontinence. *Journal of American Geriatric Society* 2001; 49(7): 892-9

- *Handbook of Geriatric Nursing.* Springhouse, PA: Springhouse Corp., 1999.

- Institute of Medicine. *To Err is Human: Building a Safer Health System.* Washington: National Academy Press; 1999.

- Johnson, ST. From incontinence to confidence. *American Journal of Nursing* 2000; 100(2): 69-74.

- King, MB, Tinetti, ME. Falls in community dwellings of older Americans. *Journal American Geriatric Society* 1995; 43(10): 1146-54.

- Kirkwood, TB, Austad, SN. Why do we age? *Nature.* 2000; 408:233-238.

- Kulpa, P. Conservative treatment of urinary stress incontinence. *Physician Sportsmedicine.* 1996; 24(7): 51-61.

- Lilley, MD. Postprandial blood pressure changes in the elderly. *Journal of Gerontologic Nursing.* 1997; 12:17-25.

- Matteson, MA. *Gerontological Nursing: Concepts and Practice*, 2nd ed. Philadelphia, PA: W.B. Saunders Co., 1997.

- McCue, JD. The naturalness of dying. *JAMA* 1995; 273(13): 1039-43.

- Pearson, LJ, editor. *Nurse Practitioner's Drug Handbook.* 3rd ed. Springhouse PA: Springhouse, 2002.

- Pelletier, K. *The Best Alternative Medicine.* New York, NY: Simon and Schuster; 2000.

- Seidel, H, et al. *Mosby's Guide to Physical Examination*, 5th ed. St. Louis, MO., Mosby Yearbook, 2003.

- Szarka, L.,et al. Diagnosing Gastroesophageal Reflux Disease, *Mayo Clinic Proceedings.*2001;76(1): 97-101.

Suggested Reading Materials

These books will provide you with additional information and clarification. If your local library does not have access to these books, call the local hospital. Most hospitals have staff and patient education libraries. Hospital libraries have access to the most current medical information.

- Beers, MH, Berkow, R. *The Merck Manual of Geriatrics.* 3rd ed. West Point, PA: Merck Research Laboratories; 2000.

- *Facts and Trends: the assisted living sourcebook.* Washington, DC: National Center for Assisted Living; 2001.

- *Handbook of Geriatric Nursing.* Springhouse, PA: Springhouse Corp., 1999.

- Matteson, MA. *Gerontological Nursing: Concepts and Practice*, 2nd ed. Philadelphia, PA: W.B. Saunders Co., 1997.

- Pearson, LJ, editor. *Nurse Practitioner's Drug Handbook.* 3rd ed. Springhouse PA: Springhouse, 2002.

- Pelletier, K. *The Best Alternative Medicine.* New York, NY: Simon and Schuster; 2000.

0-595-31168-7